Secrets of Italian Self-Care

A Guide to a Great Life of Health, Wellness, and
Longevity From a Country That Has It So You Can Live
the Life Too

Dr. Eugene Antenucci

For my grandfather Eugene Pasquini, who came to the United States at the age of 18 from Tuscany during hard times but never left Italy behind. He shared his soul with me, and his home in Lucca became mine forever. My best friend growing up, my mentor in so many ways, and my namesake. Grazie.

The Secrets of Italian Self Care

A Guide to a Great Life of Health, Wellness, and Longevity From a Country That Has It So You Can Live the Life Too

Dr. Eugene Antenucci

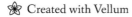 Created with Vellum

Introduction

La Dolce Vita—The Sweet Life

I hurried down the busy street, trying everything I could to hail a taxi, but no luck. My shirt stuck to my back as I hurried along Rome's vibrant streets to get to my next meeting on time. I love traveling to Italy, so when the opportunity arose to travel there for work, I grabbed it with both hands. Had I known it would be filled with meetings and seminars with hardly any time to go sightseeing, I might have reconsidered. As I rushed into the cafe, meeting another doctor to discuss a seminar opportunity, I bumped into the waiter who looked at me as if I had gone mad. I looked around the cafe, desperately searching for him. Usually, doctors were quite easy to spot, especially in the US. It's usually the one on his phone, checking his watch and signaling for the waiter to bring the bill as soon as the food is served. Yet, there I stood, no other doctor in sight. Annoyance rushed over me, frustrated that I ran all the way there and the other doctor didn't even bother to show. I was about to leave when a charming, calm, and collected man swaggered his way over, smiled, and with all the time in the world, said, "I assume you're Eugene." I nodded as he introduced himself as the doctor I was looking for. The moment we sat down at the table, I took out my laptop, ready to get right to it. He laughed charmingly and asked, "Have you had lunch yet?" Only then did I realize just how hungry I was. I shook my head, and with his Italian charm, he called the waiter over.

"What can I get you?" the waiter asked me with a thick accent. I responded by asking him what would be the quickest. My companion laughed, ordered something in Italian, and told me to close my laptop. Soon after, the waiter arrived with two glasses of red wine and a breadbasket, saying that the food was on its way. "You Americans, you are always rushing everywhere. Here, we practice the principle of *La Dolce Vita*, the sweet life." I had a look around the room and realized that everyone was extremely relaxed and not in a hurry to go anywhere. They were simply enjoying their meal and enjoying their company. On my trip to Italy, I learned a couple of valuable lessons, one of which is that I had completely forgotten how to actually live a sweet life.

Being able to slow down and actually enjoy a meal is only one of the many Italian principles that make life so sweet. In fact, the way most Italians live is naturally healthier, more enjoyable, and more peaceful. So, it came as no surprise to me when Italy got named the healthiest country in the world, where people live the longest, fullest lives. It made me reconsider the way that I do life, as well as those around me. With hustle culture, busy schedules, and increasing living costs, it's hard to sometimes just switch off and live the sweet life. I speak out of personal experience when I say that I often feel guilty when I take a couple of moments just to breathe and relax. By the end of the day, most of us fall onto the bed, completely exhausted, yet totally unaware of the life that passed us by that day. We don't stop to smell the flowers anymore, and in my opinion, it's time we get that back and start living as the Italians do.

Perhaps you feel overworked, anxious, or struggling with your health. Maybe you simply feel unsatisfied and are looking for a new way of life. Well, either way, you're in the right place. In this book, we're learning how to live *La Dolce Vita*. We're going to dissect, inspect, and apply the aspects of Italian culture that help them to live longer, healthier, and happier lives. You might wonder why the Italians and not another culture. Well, simply because the Italians have proven over decades and decades that their way of living works! They're set apart from the rest of the world because they do things differently and, most of the time, much slower than what we're used to. They prioritize rest, family, culture, religion, love, and cuisine. They show their passions, express their feelings, and put relaxation at the top of their list. And as a result, they seem to live much longer than most of us do.

If this is your first time reading a book of mine, welcome! My name is Dr. Eugene Antenucci, and I have been a health-care provider since 1983. I've conducted many seminars internationally and have a passion for nutrition and wellness. I also host a television series, *The Good Life*, with my gorgeous wife, Karina. My children might roll their eyes at me when I say this, but I truly believe that I have unlocked the secrets to living a good, full, healthy life. Not because I'm particularly smart or developed some new way of living, but because I try my best to live the Italian way, right here in America, and if you allow me, I can teach you too.

On this Italian health journey, you won't find ten easy steps to unlock immortality or anything unrealistic like that. Instead, you'll find a simplified version of everything that we need to know to live life the Italian way. I want to help you as much as I can on this journey together, but at the end of the day, only you can decide whether you want to implement what you've learned. I can't make that decision for you. If I could, I would, trust me! However, I can only make that decision for myself and no one else. If you want to make sure you are prepared for what you're about to get yourself into, here's a little sneak peek of everything you'll accomplish on this journey with me.

- We'll start by exploring why Italians live longer than the rest of the world and what exactly sets them apart to improve longevity.
- We'll discover the meaning of blue zones, more specifically, where they are and what they all have in common.
- Together, we'll explore the Mediterranean diet as a way of living and how the Italians make use of the Mediterranean diet regularly.
- We'll discuss Italian food culture, including what makes it so unique and what we can learn from it.
- Then, we'll start to look at the slow food movement, along with practical examples of how we can incorporate it into our lives.
- We'll explore the role that family plays in Italian culture and how family can contribute to better health and well-being.
- Of course, we can't talk about health and ignore the role of fitness and exercise. We'll discover how Italy incorporates fitness and socializing.
- We'll also explore the Italian spirit of community, religion, and art and how all of these can contribute to a better lifestyle.

- We'll discuss some of the easiest, yummiest recipes that will boost your health while helping you to live more freely.
- Finally, we'll put it all together and create an action plan to live life to the fullest and live the Italian way!

Are you ready to discover your *La Dolce Vita*? Don't worry, I'll be with you every step of the way. Remember, this isn't homework. This isn't a must-do-or-else kind of self-help book. This is fun! It's exploring a new way of life that will ultimately provide you with more fun, more health, and more joy.

Let's learn how to live the Italian way!

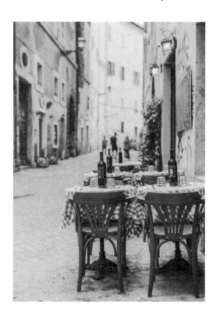

Chapter 1
The Longevity of Italians

Finché c'è vita, c'è speranza—As long as there is life, there is hope

W hen I started researching the Italian way of living, there was one important question I needed to answer: Do they really live longer than the rest of the world? In the healthcare world, it's common knowledge to know they live longer than the rest of the world, so I thought perhaps it was just a silly misconception or something true 100 years ago, but no more. So, with this question in mind, I started doing my research. I'm happy to announce that I got an answer and some other incredible facts!

Italians do live longer than most of the rest of the world. In 2020, they were ranked 6th in the world, while the US. was ranked number 46th—quite a big difference, indeed (*Why Do Italians Live So Long?* 2019). In fact, the record of the oldest living person was an Italian woman, Emma Martina Luigia Morano, who was born in 1899 and lived until 2017 (Hengel, 2017). Yes, that's right, that's 117 years! Of course, genetics play a huge role in longevity, but it's also not the only contributor. Mrs. Morano wasn't the only exception, though. In 2018, a study was conducted in Italy, using only people ages 105 and up. The study had a total of 3,836 participants, which is extraordinary! Since 2020, things have changed dramatically. Italy is no longer ranked 6th but at the top with a golden medal around its boot. That's right, Italy was crowned the healthiest country in the world in 2023, with a health score of 72.15 out of 100. To put it into perspective, the country that is considered the second healthiest, Singapore, has a score of 67.22, quite a bit below Italy (Brown, 2022).

All of this information is good and well, but it actually confirms only one thing: We need this book more than ever! We need to learn what we can from the Italians and start living in such a way as soon as possible. In this chapter, we'll look at why Italy is considered the healthiest country, according to researchers and other healthcare professionals. We need to know why if we want to copy what they're doing from our own corners of the world. We'll also zoom in a little closer and look at which Italian cities are the healthiest and why that is the case.

Why Do Italians Live Longer?

When the general health rankings are allocated to a country, a lot of research goes into it to ensure that it's accurate. *The Bloomberg Global Health Index* looks at life expectancy and the causes of death in different countries but also considers health risks, such as high blood pressure, obesity, and cholesterol. It also considers environmental factors such as carbon emissions and access to drinking water. So, it can be trusted when it claims that Italy is #1. Upon closer inspection, we see that most young Italians are in much better condition than those in other countries such as the UK and the US. Young Italians have better cholesterol levels and blood pressure, as well as better overall mental health (Hutt, 2017). But why is that the case? What makes Italians so much healthier than the rest of the world? Well, these are the reasons why!

- **The Diet**

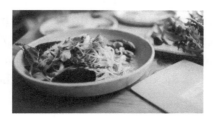

One of the biggest reasons for this incredible health difference lies in the diets that these different countries maintain. While in the US, we live on carbs and fast food, especially when we're young and hustling, in Italy, even the younger generations implement a Mediterranean diet into their daily lives. A Mediterranean diet is filled with fresh vegetables, fish, lean meats, and olive oil.

You might think that a diet can't play such a big role, but you would be mistaken. Circulatory disease is the #1 cause of global deaths, and in Italy, it's almost non-existent. That's due to their diet. Two things really stand out when you look at the Italian diet:

- Their love for fresh and local produce.
- Their preference for olive oil over animal fat.

Especially in smaller towns and villages in Italy, people prefer to shop at small businesses and family-run butchers and bakeries. This translates to a marked difference in locals' health since the food comes from their own lands. Not only does this mean that food is fresher, but it also contains more vitamins and fewer harmful pesticides and chemicals (*Why Do Italians Live So Long?* 2019). These fresh products also taste better, which is why Italians consume such large quantities of fruit and vegetables. Olive oil, in itself, has a lot of incredible benefits, which is why it plays such a big role in the Mediterranean diet. Olive oil has been shown to have a direct effect on increasing longevity, and it also decreases the risk of diabetes and heart disease (*Why Do Italians Live So Long?* 2019). For Italians, olive oil is the dressing of choice, and they have it with almost every meal.

- ### Drinking Habits

Another reason why Italians are healthier than the rest of the world is due to their drinking habits. Alcohol consumption is responsible for 2.8 million premature deaths per year (*Why Do Italians Live So Long?* 2019). Heavy drinking reduces your life expectancy by five years, so what do Italians drink? Well, they drink wine, but in moderation. They believe that a small amount of red wine a day fights off cardiovascular disease due to the antioxidants in the wine. Red wine is also the least harmful type of alcohol, making it the preferred choice at dinner. Italians mostly drink with their food, which also minimizes the harmful effects on the body. Some Italians are even known to dilute their wine to prevent over-consumption. This is especially popular among the older generations. Italy has a very low prevalence of binge drinking, especially when you compare Italian young adults with young adults from other countries (*Why Do Italians Live So Long?* 2019). The other drinking habit that contributes to their healthy lifestyle is the fact that they drink a lot of water. Italians don't drink a lot of juice or soft drinks. They'd rather stick with their water during the day.

- **The Weather**

Italians are also believed to live longer due to their weather. Italians enjoy mostly sunny weather throughout the year, with very low levels of precipitation. Since their weather is mostly sunny, it contributes to them favoring physical activity, which contributes to their longevity. When temperatures remain between 68–77°F, it allows us to feel at our best since it doesn't require us to thermoregulate. Thermoregulation is when your body shivers or sweats to maintain a better temperature, which completely depletes your energy. Italians spend a lot of time outdoors, mainly to see friends or to go for a walk together (*Why Do Italians Live So Long?* 2019). Being in the sun also gives Italians more vitamin D, improving their bone density and immune system. All of these elements together contribute to better health and longevity.

Good weather also contributes to better mental health. Sunlight boosts serotonin production, positively affecting appetite, sleep, learning, memory, and mood. When you don't get enough sun, you can suffer from a seasonal affective disorder, where your mood highly depends on the weather you're experiencing. Strong sunlight leads to better sleep since it contributes to better sleep-wake patterns. The better sleep you get, the more beneficial it is for your mental and physical health.

- **The Relaxed Schedule**

As I discovered that day in the cafe in Rome, Italians have a more relaxed pace of life, contributing to lower stress levels. Stress can severely shorten life expectancy, and due to how Italians spend their time, it's clear why they are so relaxed. When you compare how Italians and Americans spend their time, you find that Americans spend almost twice as much time working than Italians do, while Italians spend more time eating and seeing friends and family (*Why Do Italians Live So Long?* 2019). While many in the US get stuck in hustle culture, Italians find it much easier to balance their work and personal life since that is what is being prioritized.

But are all Italians really this healthy, or are there one or two small towns that influenced these statistics? There's only one way to find out!

Where Do Italians Live The Longest?

It's safe to assume that, in general, Italians live longer than the rest of the world. However, some Italians live longer than others. Obviously, we're not counting those who die from accidents or other ailments but based on average life expectancy. Four places in Italy are particularly well-known for their healthy residents, but do they live longer for the same reasons, or do some of these villages have other secrets that can unlock the mystery of aging? Let's have a closer look at these locales and their long-living citizens.

1. Sardinia

Sardinia is an Italian island in the Mediterranean. It's known for its gorgeous coastline and pristine waters. However, many claim that Sardinia is the fountain of youth that many people have sought. Interestingly enough, while all around the world, women are known to outlive men, in Sardinia, this doesn't seem to be the case. When looking at the data per capita, Sardinia has nearly ten times more people 100 years of age or older than the US. Many men and women in Sardinia live into their 90s and 100s (Tucci, 2020). The Sardinia lifestyle highly contributes to this statistic, as they are very active. It's very common to walk a couple of miles a day doing common errands and tasks, and men would often walk up steep mountains through the pastures as they worked as goat shepherds. The ones who can't climb mountains anymore stay active and mobile by working in the garden, cooking, and cleaning. Most Sardinians have their own backyard garden filled with fresh produce for daily consumption (Tucci, 2020). Barley is about 50% of their intake, and they don't consider meat an essential staple to every meal. Of course, Sardinians also drink a lot of water and consume large amounts of olive oil. In Sardinia, people drink wine called Cannonau (Tucci, 2020). Cannonau wine has anti-inflammatory benefits and very high levels of antioxidants.

Sardinians believe heavily in the spirit of community and not going through life alone. Family and community traditions are incredibly important for Sardinians; they value relationships above all else. Even though Sardinians have strong work ethics, they enjoy a relaxed work-life balance and experience little stress. Sardinians love what they do and continue working for as long as possible, not just until it's time to retire. Laughing and spending time together with friends is something that Sardinians do regularly. It's very rare to find someone in Sardinia in a foul mood. They also have a lot of respect for their elders, and age is something that is celebrated as wisdom. Elders aren't placed in nursing homes but form part of the community, live under the same roof as their families, and remain active for as long as possible (Tucci, 2020).

2. Campodimele

Campodimele is a southern village in Italy. People here live to an exceptional age, almost 30 years longer than the average Italian elsewhere. The people in Campodimele pride themselves on living longer and remaining healthy in mind and body as they age (Britannica, n.d.). In 1987, a former police officer in Rome published a book filled with astonishing findings about this mountain village. He researched their longevity and the contributing factors that made this small village so healthy and mobile. Eventually, he became the mayor of Campodimele.

Campodimele is a farming village, and five generations are often found working side-by-side in the fields. They live off what they yield from the field, often consuming large amounts of fresh vegetables. Scalonga is a type of onion that can only be found in Campodimele, and it contains substances that aid in digestion and strengthen the immune system (Britannica, n.d.). In the village, people eat very little meat but consume a lot of olive oil and homemade bread. The sprightly villagers have virtually no experience with heart disease (Britannica, n.d.). In Campodimele, villagers drink a glass of red wine with every meal. The small village has a population of 800 people, and over 120 of these people are over the age of 80.2.

3. Acciaroli

Only a short drive from the Amalfi Coast, you'll find a beautiful, small village filled with many healthy older people. Acciaroli is a seaside town, extremely charming and filled with rich culture. Alan Maisel, an American cardiologist, did a study on this town and found that of the around 1,000 residents in Acciaroli, 300 of those live to be over 100 years old (McGuire, 2017). In Acciaroli, people enjoy seasonal vegetables and olive oil, just like in the other villages, but there's one thing that's different: rosemary. Rosemary grows naturally throughout the village, and they use it in almost every meal. The health benefits of this plant are undeniable and probably a big contributor to their amazing health and longevity. In Acciaroli, villagers walk every day. They very rarely use any other mode of transportation and use their feet to get where they want to be. Naturally, this active lifestyle contributes to their health and wellness. They also believe in strong family ties, and many families who live in Acciaroli have been there for generations.

4. **Molochio**

Molochio is another small village on Italy's southern hilly coastline. Approximately 2,000 people live in this small village, and a large proportion of these people are over 100 years old. A National Geographic reporter asked Salvatore Caruso, a 106-year-old habitant of Molochio, what his secret to living longer is. He proudly answered, *"No bacco, no tobacco, no venere!"* which roughly translates to, "No drinking, no smoking, and no women" (Ledsom, 2022). Upon further investigation, Caruso also said that he had lived mostly on beans and figs and rarely ate red meat. Another 103-year-old who lived in Molochio echoed what Caruso said. He said, *"Poco, ma tutto,"* which means "A little bit, but of everything." Many people living in Molochio claimed that they fasted for long periods when they were little due to poverty. Fasting led to stronger immunities and better resilience. In Molochio, people also value a more relaxed way of life and don't believe in stressing over material possessions (Ledsom, 2022).

Just by examining these four towns in Italy, we can already start to see a pattern. However, before we jump to conclusions and decide what we need to do to be healthier and live longer, perhaps, we should quickly look at other healthy countries and what they have in common with Italy.

What Do Some of the Healthiest Countries Have in Common?

When we look at the countries that are considered healthy, there are a few things that they all have in common. Four things, in particular, stand out when we compare other healthy countries with Italy.

1. **Walking**

Everyone walks everywhere in countries that are considered healthier. A whopping 37% of Spaniards walk to work every day, while less than 6% of Americans walk to work, or anywhere for that matter (Miles, 2020). Even as we look at the small villages in Italy with the oldest people, it's clear that walking and being active play a large role. Very few people in Italy and these other healthy countries "exercise." They don't go for a run or swim laps in the ocean, and you would very rarely find anyone hitting the gym; instead, they all maintain active lifestyles. Especially in the smaller towns, very few people have office jobs, and since everyone walks to the markets and back on a daily basis, they get in more steps than most of us who go to the gym. Since most of the people living in small villages maintain their own gardens, they are generally more active than those in more modern societies who just get Uber Eats every night. Perhaps we should take this as a hint. Maybe we should start worrying less about abs and thighs and focus more on walking and being life fit.

2. **Food**

Italy is not the only country that predominantly makes use of the Mediterranean diet. Most countries that are considered the healthiest eat similar diets to the Italians. Most healthy countries focus on many fresh products that are maintained locally, and they maintain a diet filled with vegetables, olive oil, and fish. In many of these countries, even the "fast food" places offer healthy alternatives. While in the States, it's the norm to eat a lot of takeout food which usually consists of a lot of carbs and very few vegetables; however, in these other countries like Italy, having junk food is the exception, not the rule. Even their pizza and pasta are considered healthier due to the local wheat and vegetables they use and not being fried or smothered in copious amounts of cheese. These healthier countries have another food-related similarity: fresh water. Having fresh water that's easily accessible contributes highly to the overall health of people, and it also influences how much water people consume. You will naturally consume less water if you don't have access to fresh water. However, if fresh drinking water is the norm over soft drinks, then you'll drink more water and fewer soft drinks.

3. Friends and Family

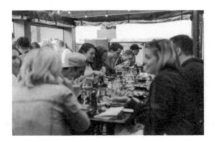

We previously learned that Italians spend a lot of time socializing. Well, they're not the only ones. In fact, most countries considered healthy prioritize socializing and spending time with friends and family. On a trip to Lucca, Italy, I was astonished at how many people were seen sitting and chatting with one another. While in most places in the United States, we're used to an "avoid eye contact" approach to people, it was quite the opposite in Lucca. In fact, in the evenings, certain roads would be closed to all cars, and tables were set up right on the streets so that people could catch up with one another. Spending time with friends and family contributes greatly to your mental health. Spending time with the ones you love is not seen as a weekend occasion in these countries but rather an everyday occurrence.

4. Healthcare

The last element that most of these countries have in common is access to healthcare. When you have access to good healthcare, it's obvious that you'll most likely be healthier. When healthcare services are something that you don't have access to, or something that's too expensive for you to consider, chances are that you won't go for regular check-ups. Healthcare, unfortunately, is not something that the everyday person can necessarily change since it's not in our control. However, we can still try our best to ensure that we get checked regularly and reach out to others in need.

There you have it, the four things that most healthy countries have in common. It makes you think about the way you live, doesn't it? Well, that's good. It means that you're starting to think about the different principles that you'll be able to implement going forward. Don't run ahead too far; we still have lots to learn on this journey. In the next chapter, we'll look at other healthy countries, including Italy, to understand blue zones.

Chapter 2
The Blue Zones

La vita è bella—Life is beautiful

When Gianni Pes and Michel Poulain identified Sardinia as a region where people grow old and live happily, they drew a circle on the map around the area and named it the *blue zone*. As their study grew, they identified other regions with the same effect as Sardinia, which led to the term "blue zones." Blue zones are, in short, regions in the world where people live longer than the average person. As we saw in the previous chapter, most of these blue zones have similar lifestyles. As of yet, there are only five blue zones across the globe, with many initiatives to transform other regions into blue zones as well. While many believe that good genetics is the cause of a long life, genetics can't take credit for the whole thing. Things like diet, exercise, and mental health play a large role in longevity and a fulfilled life.

In this chapter, we'll look at the five blue zones in detail and discuss why they are so extraordinary. Once we've discussed them, we'll have a clearer picture of what it takes to be considered a blue zone. Ultimately, we want to turn your life into a small blue zone. We might not be able to control an entire country or region, but we can control our own surroundings and way of living. Are you ready to make your own life beautiful and learn what it takes to be a blue zone? Then, let's get right into it. The five blue zones are:

- Loma Linda, California, United States
- Nicoya Peninsula, Costa Rica
- Ikaria, Greece
- Okinawa, Japan
- Sardinia, Italy

Loma Linda

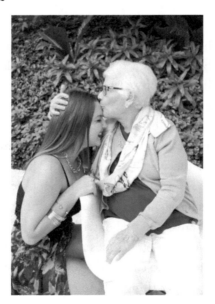

It surprised many when a city in the United States made the cut to be identified as a blue zone since America is known for many things, but certainly not its health. However, Loma Linda might just be the blueprint for the rest of the states. What makes Loma Linda such an interesting study is the fact that almost its entire population are Seventh-day Adventists. With a population of roughly 24,000 people, Loma Linda is home to a large Seventh-day Adventist community, with a third of the people participating in this religion. Researchers have found that these Seventh-day Adventists live approximately a decade longer than non-religious people in Northern America (Spector, 2019). The people who live in Loma Linda are considered the oldest living people in the entire United States. What makes Loma Linda stand out from other blue zones is the fact that it's not geographically isolated. It's not on an island or far from other civilizations, and Loma Linda proves it doesn't have to be.

You might wonder, so what does their religion have to do with it? Seventh-day Adventists adopt a healthful diet and abstain from "unclean foods," as their scripture identifies. Unclean food includes alcohol, tobacco, and the use of recreational drugs. Many Seventh-day Adventists are also vegetarians and eat a diet consisting mostly of fruits and vegetables. The church in Loma Linda was founded in 1840 and flourished due to its dedicated members. Even today, the community of the church is strong and at the core of the blue zone (Buettner, 2008a). The people of Loma Linda also live active lifestyles. There seems to be another secret to the success of Loma Linda: rest.

Most Seventh-day Adventists in Loma Linda switch off completely every Friday evening after work or school. Work, books, and other responsibilities are put away and placed on hold. They also turn off other distractions, such as the TV or radio, and rather spend their Friday evenings singing alongside their neighbors and participating in the Sabbath (Mikhail, 2023). On Saturdays, they attend church and volunteer in the community. They often participate in activities with other families, usually something outdoors, like cycling or walking. On Saturday evenings, different families would come together to enjoy games, eat potluck-style dinner, and then have a sundown worship session (Mikhail, 2023). It's almost like a mini vacation, where, for at least 48 hours, you are completely switched off and take a break. Unplugging allows them to de-stress, let go of the week's madness, and remember what is important in life.

The name of this city actually translates to "beautiful hill," and they have been named one of the top high-performing healthcare providers in the country. Dr. Ellsworth Wareham is the perfect example of this. As a resident of Loma Linda, he was a cardiothoracic surgeon, and he practiced medicine until he was 95 years old. While working hard every weekend, he switched off, focused on his family and friends, and mowed the lawn himself. He lived a vegan lifestyle and died at the age of 104, still mobile and active (Mikhail, 2023). Unlike other blue zones, Loma Linda isn't known for its aesthetic look. It's less about the place itself but rather about the people and the life-style they follow. This is good news for the rest of the world! It means that you don't have to live on an exotic island before you start living life as if you're in a blue zone.

Nicoya Peninsula

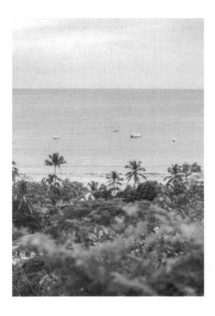

In the mountains of Costa Rica, you'll find the rural landscapes of the Nicoya Peninsula. Unlike tourist-driven Costa Rican areas near the beach, these rural areas are deep in the mountains. It is right here that you'll find another blue zone containing some of the people with the longest lifespans in the world (Pitura, 2021). The people in the Nicoya Peninsula live vibrant lives that appear almost stuck in a time capsule. In these rural areas, monkeys, parrots, and other wildlife live in tandem with humans, and they rise together at the crack of dawn. The people in Nicoya make use of horses as their mode of transportation, and they use oxcarts to transport things from point A to point B. As crazy as it might seem at first to be so far removed from modern inventions, it also means that they are removed from modern stresses. The natives in Nicoya live according to *plan de vida,* which means to live with a reason. Even those aged 90 years and older still live a life where they fulfill a purpose. Instead of retiring and simply waiting for life to be over, they focus on family, being active, and supporting their neighbors all throughout their lives (Buettner, 2008b).

Everyone in the Nicoya Peninsula has a purpose. Family, friends, and community are high on their priority list, which provides them with an additional sense of purpose. Many people walk to their family members and friends on a daily basis to share, love, and laugh together. It provides them with a reason to live and a reason to be happy. They find another sense of purpose in their faith. Most people in these rural areas are Catholic and take their spiritual life very seriously. They believe that their connection to the spiritual world helps them to live longer. Nicoyan centenarians live mostly with their families, and retirement homes are very rarely a thing. Due to this, most of the Nicoyans work hard physically, no matter their age. They find joy in completing daily tasks.

Nicoyans also get a lot of exposure to the sun, especially during the dry months, which lasts from December to May. During these months, a majority of Nicoyan people take up an outdoor lifestyle, where they'll spend as much time as possible outside. This provides them with an abundance of vitamin D, contributing to better body function. Nicoyans will often be spotted outside, sharing dinner with each other or walking together to local markets.

One of the most remarkable things regarding the Nicoyan lifestyle is their diet. Nicoyans eat mainly unprocessed, wholesome food, such as squash, rice, beans, and corn. They grow most of their food at home and only eat meat once or twice weekly (Pitura, 2021). They also have larger meals during the day and eat smaller meals at dinner, which contributes to better digestion and lower body fat. They drink a lot of water, and the water in this area is especially strong. Strong water refers to the amount of calcium and magnesium that can be found in the water. Since their water is mineral-rich, there are almost no signs of osteoporosis or heart disease.

Nicoya is the perfect example that you don't need riches to live a healthier, longer life. It would appear to be quite the opposite. Many of the changes required to build more blue zones appear to be a virtue of less and not more.

Ikaria

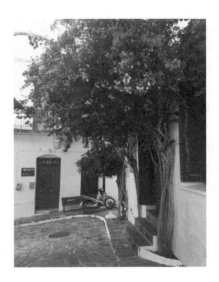

This tiny island in Greece is often referred to as "the island where people forget to die." This small island is rich with history and people who live long and happy lives. It's said that one in three Ikarians make it into their 90s (*Ikaria, Greece*, n.d.). This outcropping of the Aegean Sea has been the target of many Persian, Roman, and Turk invasions. These invasions forced residents to move inland. As a result, the isolated culture formed rich family virtues and traditions and promoted longevity (*Ikaria, Greece*, n.d.). One of the most interesting things about Ikarians is that they are almost completely free from dementia. Once again, the longevity in Ikaria isn't due to only one factor but rather several small things working together in the favor of the people.

Ikarians are known to be extremely social people. Elisa Sinadinou traveled to Ikaria in 2018 to explore the culture for herself. Her ancestors were Ikarians, but she had never been there before 2018. The first thing she noted was how friendly everyone was. Despite thousands of tourists flooding the streets of Ikaria, the Ikarians are friendly and social toward one another and outsiders. In fact, many would invite you into their homes for coffee, olives, and cheese. They are also proud of their creative work and would often invite you to appreciate their paintings or crochet work (Sinadinou, 2018). She noted that most Ikarians look at least a decade younger than their actual age and are very sharp mentally and physically.

Ikaria is named after the mythological figure Icarus, the man who ignored his father's warning about flying too close to the sun. Eventually, he did, and it melted the wax in his wings. He ended up falling and was washed up dead on the shores. Although ancient lore connects Ikaria with youthful reckless-ness, the town of Ikaria is quite the opposite, filled with centen-nials who carry wisdom. These longevity claims aren't new. In fact, in 1678, a writer named Iosif Georgirinis published a book where he attributed the Ikarians' longevity to their fresh water and diet (Sinadinou, 2018). The Ikarians have a simple way of living, although tiring in their own way. They have a laid-back attitude and strive to live stress-free. Christodoulos Xenakis, a neurologist and native to Ikaria, is in charge of organizing the yearly Ikaria Senior Regatta, which is a sailing competition for anyone over 70 years old. This is just one of the many ways that Ikarians celebrate age and do not write them off as being "finished."

The Ikarians strongly believe in a daily siesta, which is

what we would call a nap (Sinadinou, 2018). Allowing for rest in the middle of the day is a virtue this island lives by. This is part of their secret to a longer life. Instead of seeing rest as useless and time-wasting, they prioritize rest and respect each other's resting periods. Being able to rest is highly understated, especially in modern societies. Being able to rest is allowing yourself a little bit of a recharge before continuing the rest of your day with energy and kindness. It's impossible to spend evenings socializing if you are too tired from your day's work.

The Ikarian diet is typical of the Mediterranean-style diet. However, it's more than just a lifestyle choice for the Ikarians, it's simply what they have available. The Ikarians mostly grow their gardens and share what they have with each other. They don't consume a lot of meat and use homemade olive oil. Many Ikarians also make their own cheese, and they enjoy strong wine. Besides wine, they also enjoy herbal teas with family and friends (*Ikaria, Greece*, n.d.). They often make herbal teas with rosemary, sage, oregano, and lemon beebrush. They sweeten their tea with honey and drink it at breakfast and sometimes before bed. The Ikarians also have a good understanding of the different types of herbs and their special properties. If you want to relax, they'll brew you a blend of aloe, basil, honey, and wine. They have another secret to their happiness: trivoli, an herb with the same qualities as Viagra (Sinadinou, 2018).

Besides their healthy eating habits and hospitality, Ikarians also maintain an active lifestyle. They often walk long distances to visit people and to go to the market. They also maintain their own gardens and work actively to keep themselves mobile. They move without considering it as exercise, simply seeing it as their way of life. Many Ikarians walk with their friends during the evenings or walk to other family members to take them fruit and vegetables. One Ikarian man gave Elisa (2018) the following advice that we can all live by:

Eat half as much, walk twice as much, laugh three times as much, and love without bounds.

Perhaps this is advice we should all take, regardless of our zone.

Okinawa

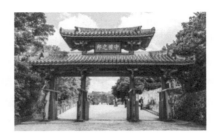

The island at the southern end of Japan is known for its longevity, especially among the women. Once called the land of immortals, Okinawa is known to have less cancer, lower cases of heart disease, and almost no cases of dementia (Buettner, 2008c). Okinawa has been extensively researched since 1975 after they found that Okinawans lived almost a decade longer than the average person. Okinawa isn't a wealthy island, and they've endured many hardships to cultivate a lifestyle that promotes longer lives.

One of the main things that Okinawans embrace is something called *moai*. Your *moai* is your circle of friends that you have for your entire life. They are the people you grow old with and the ones who stand by you, regardless of your life season. Your *moai* provides you with a secure social network that installs a sense of safety and emotional support within your life. It actively removes the fear of rejection and loneliness, which contributes to a much better mental state. Having a *moai* is like knowing you have people in your corner who will never leave you and will always be there to support you (Buettner, 2008c).

Another thing that Okinawans do is something called *ikigai*. They believe that everyone is called to embrace their *ikigai*, which is your purpose in life (Katira, 2022). Your *ikigai* is the reason you get out of bed in the morning and why you keep going regardless of your age. Your *ikigai* isn't necessarily your job but your passions and hobbies. The Okinawans believe that everyone should have clear goals and actively work towards them to feel like they have a purpose in life (Katira, 2022). They believe that without a sense of purpose, you will die. The idea is that with clear goals and responsibilities, you'll be more driven and feel like you are being useful, which contributes to longevity.

In Okinawa, the diet is plant-based beginning from childhood. This includes a lot of stir-fry, sweet potatoes, and tofu that is high in nutrients. They also live by the 80% rule, which says that you should stop eating when you feel 80% full to avoid overeating and binge eating. Okinawans also incorporate a lot of Goya, which is filled with antioxidants and aids in keeping blood sugar low. Their diet also consists of a lot of soy and miso soup. Tofu is known to protect women against breast cancer and to guard them against heart attacks (Katira, 2022). Their fermented soy foods also contribute to their intestinal health and offer them nutritional benefits.

Okinawans love to garden, and almost everyone has their own garden where they plant vegetables, fruits, and herbs. Some Okinawans dedicate their garden to be used as medical gardens where they plant herbs that contain medicinal qualities. You'll often find mugwort, turmeric, and ginger in their gardens, which protects them against illnesses (Buettner, 2008c). Gardening also keeps them active, which helps with circulation and improved health. Besides gardening, Okinawans walk everywhere they need to go, and they often walk socially to catch up with friends and family. Their homes have very limited furniture, and residents often take meals while sitting on the floor or on tatami mats. Even old people have to get up and down from the ground several times a day, which builds muscle and balance.

The last thing that is so wonderful about Okinawans is their attitude. They have a hardship-tempered attitude which helps them to push through difficulties while enjoying the simple things that every day has to offer. Older Okinawans believe you should surround yourself with younger people to remain young, so you'll often find groups of people chatting, varying over generations. This serves as a good reminder for all of us not to push older people out of society but to supply them with a purpose.

Sardinia

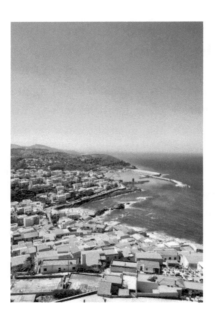

We already spoke about beautiful Sardinia in the previous chapter since it is a region in Italy. This cluster of villages was the world's first blue zone and the start of all this wonderful discovery and life-changing knowledge. What we can learn from Sardinia is that a good community goes a long way. Since Sardinians highly value their traditions, they stay close to friends and family, which highly contributes to their longevity. As with all four other blue zones, Sardinians eat a Mediterranean-style diet and stay active as an integral part of their lifestyle.

So, what can we conclude from these five blue zones? Is there something we can learn and hold on to while we continue on this journey and incorporate healthy habits? There sure is! After inspecting the five blue zones, researchers created *the power nine,* which is a list of nine things that you can learn from these blue zones to make your own life a blue zone. Let's have a closer look.

The Power Nine

I'm sure as you read through the five blue zones, you were starting to see many similarities. Well, so did the researchers, who created a list of nine characteristics each blue zone shares and called it the power nine. The *power nine* is the beginning of the rest of this journey. It sets the foundation for what each of us needs to incorporate and change in our lives to live healthier and live the Italian way. Let's briefly look at each of the power nine to determine where we want to start with our own change.

1. Move Naturally

People who live in blue zones aren't weekend warriors (Chandler, 2022). They live in an environment that encourages movement throughout the day through gardening, housework, and their terrain. They move around all day without the luxury of mechanical conveniences. So, start taking the stairs and turn your backyard into a garden.

2. Purpose

The blue zones emphasize the importance of living meaningful lives by committing to a goal, ideal, or cause. There is a common belief in something bigger and that every person has a purpose until the day they die. Your purpose doesn't have an expiration date. You are still considered a valuable member of society even as you get older. Having a sense of purpose will help you to get out of bed in the morning and make the most out of your day.

3. Downshift

Blue zones are serious about their downtime. While some de-stress by praying and participating in religious activities, others make sure to nap or spend time with family (Chandler, 2022). The world is getting increasingly more stressful by the day, and if we don't take care of our stress on a daily basis, it becomes overwhelming. Taking time to de-stress is not something that should only be considered once a week, but rather something that should be implemented daily.

4. The 80% Rule

The American lifestyle tends to be filled with large meals in the evenings and eating until you can hardly move. While eating until you feel full and satisfied is important, you shouldn't overeat on a daily or even weekly basis. The blue zones make use of an 80% rule, where they stop eating before they feel overly full. They also prioritize having smaller dinners and eating their larger meals during the day. Many Americans eat small things that they can grab on the go during the day and leave their biggest meal for late at night. However, there are many health benefits to having your last meal at least three hours before you go to bed.

5. Plant-Based

Blue zones all love their veggies. Beans, such as fava, soy, and lentils, are common denominators within blue zone diets (Chandler, 2022). Most blue zones eat mostly vegetables, and meat is rarely on the menu, with studies showing that have found that for most, meat is eaten five times a month. This is quite different from the traditional Western diet, with meat usually being the center of the meal and vegetables only there to support it.

6. Wine

All the blue zones except Loma Linda partake in a happy hour. Daily at 5 p.m., they will have some wine. The key lies in moderate consumption and not getting drunk. Sardinia is known for its Cannonau wine, which has three times more antioxidants than other wines (Chandler, 2022). Drinking wine is usually accompanied by food, and the goal is not to overindulge. It is seen as part of the meal and part of the daily routine. Of course, since Loma Linda are Seventh-day Adventists, they abstain from drinking wine.

7. Belonging

When you feel like you belong somewhere, it improves

your longevity. In a study, 263 centenarians who live in blue zones were interviewed, and from the entire group, only five weren't part of a faith-based community. When you are part of a faith, you get a sense of belonging among other believers and within the faith community. Often centenarians also find their sense of purpose by participating in voluntary work in their faith-filled community. The blue zones strongly believe in belonging and create opportunities for older generations to belong to something, for example, the Senior Regatta sailing competition for seniors 70 and up in Ikaria!

8. Family and Friends

All five blue zones make no secret of the fact that they value spending a lot of time with friends and family. Generally, they live either with or close to family and visit almost daily. They value spending quality time together with their loved ones, and they believe that family should come before anything else. Family is prioritized first, and then the rest. Unfortunately, across the globe, this is not the case. Those we love the most are neglected in order to squeeze in some extra work or to achieve something new.

9. Right Tribe

The last of the power nine points is about finding the right tribe. When you have a strong social network, you have a better chance at longevity. In fact, social networks reinforce healthy habits, and they provide emotional support. Blue zones emphasize the importance of finding your tribe and openly testify to how their friends have saved them over the years. If you have a tribe that is there to support you and encourage you, you have found the right tribe. Okinawans are especially fond of this principle with their *"moais."* They believe in sticking together for life! What a refreshing thought to think that when you make friends, they are there for life.

Now that we've discussed the different blue zones, and we've identified the power nine tools, it's time to jump into some practical aspects of Italian health. The first thing we'll look at is diet. Take a moment to think about your daily diet. If you were to write down everything you ate this week, would it be a balanced list? Would it look good in comparison to Italians, or would you feel guilty as you try to hide another McDonald's box? Whatever the case, this is a journey, and we're all about making progress. So, let's start by making progress toward a better diet, specifically the Mediterranean diet.

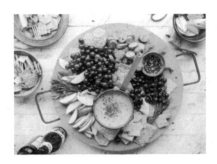

Chapter 3
The Mediterranean Diet

Buon cibo. Buon vino. Buon amici Good food. Good wine. Good friends.

The Mediterranean diet isn't a brand-new concept by any means. In fact, if you have a heart disease or some other chronic condition like high blood pressure, your doctor might have even prescribed this diet to you. The Mediterranean diet is often connected to decreasing heart disease, depression, and dementia. However, it can be beneficial even to those who don't have any chronic ailments or are at risk of heart disease. The diet in itself has changed and evolved with time. The Italian Mediterranean diet in itself looks somewhat different than the Mediterranean diet elsewhere. The Mediterranean diet was first described in the mid-20th century in Crete, Greece, and Southern Italy (The Nutrition Source, 2018). During those years, the impact the diet had on those countries was significant. With lower rates of chronic diseases and a higher quality of adult life, the diet became quite popular across the world.

Since the diet has different variations, it can get tricky to identify which foods are allowed and which aren't. Luckily, the World Health Organization released a pyramid to describe the different food groups that should be welcomed and prioritized in a Mediterranean diet. The pyramid also included daily exercise since it forms part of what makes the Mediterranean diet so efficient.

In this chapter, we'll look at what exactly it means to eat according to the Mediterranean diet. We'll explore what a Mediterranean diet looks like and what it would entail for the everyday person outside of Italy. We'll also look at the benefits of the Mediterranean diet and address some of the concerns and cons. Finally, we'll look at how the Italian Mediterranean diet differs from other Mediterranean diets. Are you ready to learn all about the diet that will change your life and your health forever? Then, without further ado, let's get right to it.

What Does a Mediterranean Diet Look Like?

As we mentioned, there are many definitions of this diet, each with its own different goals and suggestions. That's mainly because the Mediterranean diet focuses on an eating pattern and not on a strict formula or calculation. The Mediterranean diet doesn't include calorie counting or heavy restrictions. Instead of focusing on what you shouldn't be eating, this diet focuses on what you should eat (*Mediterranean Diet*, 2022). This ensures that the diet is pretty flexible and can be modified to fit everyone's personal preference while still being beneficial. You can tailor the diet to your own needs while still reaping the benefits.

The Mediterranean diet is primarily a plant-based diet. This means that it focuses on incorporating whole grains, olives, fruit, vegetables, and beans daily (The Nutrition Source,

2018). Other food groups like dairy and meat are eaten in smaller quantities, and when they are included, the focus is on adding fish and seafood before meat. The Mediterranean diet doesn't focus on portion sizes since it relies on intuitive eating. Intuitive eating involves being in touch with your body, eating until you are full, and stopping when you are no longer hungry, regardless of how much food you have left. It is up to each individual to decide exactly how much they want to eat, and it can also change depending on the season, the day, and how much physical activity they participate in that specific day.

There are a few things that make this diet stand out from other diets aside from the fact that it contributes to longevity. Let's have a look at some of these factors of the Mediterranean diet (The Nutrition Source, 2018):

- **Healthy Fats**

The Mediterranean diet places heavy emphasis on healthy fats. While other diets restrict any and all types of fats, the Mediterranean diet recommends using olive oil in your cooking, and instead of cutting out the fat in your current diet, it recommends replacing it with healthy fats such as olive oil. The diet recommends cutting out butter and margarine and replacing it with olive oil or other healthy fats, which include avocados, nuts, oily fish like salmon and sardines, and walnuts. This way, you can still eat delicious food without restricting yourself from the use of fats. Take a moment to consider your daily fat intake. Do you make use of any of these healthy fats in your daily diet? Start by adding some high-quality, organic olive oil to your shopping list and remove ultra-processed vegetable oils like canola oil from your pantry.

- **Fish as Your Main Source of Protein**

While many diets promote a higher protein intake, especially if it is accompanied by an exercise program, the Mediterranean diet is different in its approach to protein. Instead of getting protein through red meat, the Mediterranean diet encourages eating mostly fish as the source of protein. In general, the Mediterranean diet doesn't include a lot of protein. It limits poultry, eggs, and dairy use to smaller portions and only a couple of times a week. Red meat is limited to only a few times per month. The rest of the time, fish is the way to go. Adding fish to your diet might feel strange initially, especially if you're not used to cooking with fish, but it is a healthy and delicious way of ensuring a fair share of high-quality protein. The Mediterranean diet doesn't promote the use of protein boosters and additional supplements to lose weight. It's all about living naturally.

- **Water, Wine, and More Water**

Rather than juice or soft drinks, the Mediterranean diet promotes drinking a lot of water. Water is considered a daily beverage, and depending on your activity level, it is suggested to drink at least eight glasses of water a day. Water isn't the only thing you're allowed to drink, though. The Mediterranean diet encourages wine drinking with meals. The goal is not to drink so much wine that you are intoxicated. Moderation is key; hence, why it should be taken with a meal. It is for enjoyment and for health purposes that wine is included in the Mediterranean diet. Other alcohols aren't encouraged since most alcoholic beverages contain a lot of sugar. Rather stick to your water and your wine.

- **Whole Grain Is the Way to Go**

Unlike other diets, the Mediterranean diet doesn't restrict you from eating starch. Whole grains are highly encouraged and form part of daily meals. Whole grain contains more benefits than refined grains, and it can be equally as tasteful. Whole grains that are encouraged include whole wheat bread and brown rice. Whole-grain food is a great alternative, especially if you enjoy bread and pasta. Whole grains contain three parts: the bran, the germ, and the endosperm. They are high in iron, magnesium, and selenium. Whole grains can contribute to your health, and the simple act of swapping your refined grains for whole grains can prevent heart disease, cancer, and type-2 diabetes (Raman, 2018). Other examples of whole grains include oats, buckwheat, bulgur wheat, and millet.

Taking all of this into consideration, a Mediterranean diet will contain the following:

- vegetables, fruits, beans, lentils, and nuts
- whole grains, like brown rice, farro, bulgar wheat and oats
- olive oil
- fish which is high in omega-3 fatty acids
- dairy in moderation
- small amounts of red meat
- little to no sweets or sugary drinks
- wine with meals
- no processed food

Eating the Mediterranean way may feel strange at first, with sugar cravings as you detox, but the longer you stick with it, the easier it will be. When you crave something sweet, instead of avoiding the craving, have some fruits and herbal tea to scratch the itch. The goal is not to restrict yourself from eating tasty meals but rather to learn how to make sure that your meals are heathy as well as tasty.

Benefits of a Mediterranean Diet

There are many benefits to the Mediterranean diet, some slightly more obvious than others. While most people who choose the Mediterranean diet at first do so for the weight loss benefits, many experience a wide range of other benefits as soon as they start eating the Mediterranean diet. Some of the benefits are considered preventive benefits, meaning that you won't necessarily see them because it's preventing something else from showing up, like certain illnesses. Let's explore eight benefits of a Mediterranean diet, all based on studies (Salomon & Lawler, 2022).

1. Reduces the Risk of Heart Disease

The first and probably most popular benefit of a Mediter-ranean diet is the fact that it reduces the risk of heart disease. Thinking back to the blue zones, this makes sense since all the blue zones had very little to no cases of heart disease. In 2017, a study was conducted, which is known as the *Predimed* study. Researchers followed 7,000 women in Spain with type-2 diabetes who were at high risk of cardiovascular disease. These women were divided into three groups, and all of them received guidance on the Mediterranean diet. However, Group 1 was given olive oil with the instruction to consume a certain amount daily. Group 2 was given nuts to consume daily, and Group 3 wasn't given anything additional (Salomon & Lawler, 2022). The researchers found that 30% of Groups 1 and 2 showed a lower risk of heart events than the control group (Group 3). This showed that the Mediterranean diet, to its full extent, is extremely beneficial for heart health. Another study later repeated this structure to disprove the original study and found that it was, in fact, true. Eating a Mediterranean diet can quite literally save your life since it's so good for your heart.

2. Reduces the Risk of a Stroke

Since we know that the Mediterranean diet is good for your heart, thanks to the *Predimed* study, we also know that it can reduce the risk of a stroke, specifically in women. A study conducted in the United Kingdom looked at women between the ages of 40 and 77. All of the women were asked to follow a strict Mediterranean diet, and the results were fascinating. They found that the Mediterranean diet reduced their chances of having a stroke by 20% (Salomon & Lawler, 2022). When strokes do occur, those on a Mediterranean diet also have a higher chance of making a full recovery than those who aren't. So, not only does the Mediterranean diet help prevent strokes, but it also aids in the recovery of stroke patients. This is another reason why the residents of the blue zones are so healthy and why they are quick to recover after any illness.

3. Prevents Cognitive Decline

As we get older, cognitive decline is natural for most. In some cases, it can lead to dementia and Alzheimer's. The Mediterranean diet fights the decline that takes place in memory and skill with age (Salomon & Lawler, 2022). According to a doctor at the Alzheimer's Association in Chicago, Dr. Sexton says that the Mediterranean diet can reduce the risk of dementia and Alzheimer's. Cognitive decline can't really be treated or prevented in any other way, which makes the Mediterranean diet even more valuable to all ages.

Since nutrition is such an incredibly important aspect of longevity, it should be taken as seriously as preparing for your retirement in any other way. The Mediterranean diet isn't the only one that offers brain protection, but it has been tried and tested by many. A study looked at the brain scans of 70 people who had no signs of dementia and scored them closely on how their eating patterns compared to a Mediterranean diet. The ones who had little to no overlap with a Mediterranean diet showed they had lower brain energy and a bigger chance of developing dementia.

4. Weight Loss

When you follow a Mediterranean diet, you will naturally lose some weight due to the added fresh foods and reduced intake of sugar and processed foods (Salomon & Lawler, 2022). The Mediterranean diet offers a way of losing weight that is sustainable and safe without causing harm. While many other diets rely heavily on restricting certain foods, the Mediterranean diet focuses more on what to add to your diet instead of what to remove for good. Of course, the results of the Mediterranean diet for weight loss may take longer to show than those of other diets since it's done in a slower but more sustainable way. Olive oil is considered taboo by many other diets because of the belief that it works against weight loss efforts. The Mediterranean diet doesn't just help you to get rid of weight, but it also aids in keeping the weight off and maintaining a healthy balance. A recent study conducted in Israel identified 322 moderately obese, middle-aged participants. They split the group into three. Group one was asked to follow a low-fat diet, the second group was asked to follow a Mediterranean diet, and the third group was asked to follow a low-carb diet. They found that those who followed the low-fat diet lost 6.4 pounds in general, while those who followed the low-carb diet lost 10.3 pounds on average. The Mediterranean diet followers lost an average of 9.7 pounds, proving that the Mediterranean diet is highly effective for weight loss.

5. Fights Type-2 Diabetes

From previous studies, we already know that the Mediterranean diet helps those who have type-2 diabetes to fight against heart disease and strokes, but the diet can do more than that. In fact, using the participants of the *Predimed* study, researchers identified a group of 418 participants without diabetes. They followed them for four years to see whether they'd developed the disease. Amazingly, the study found that those who followed the Mediterranean diet had a 52% lower risk of getting type-2 diabetes than others (Salomon & Lawler, 2022). The reason for this is due to the low sugar intake on the Mediterranean diet. The Mediterranean diet ultimately helps ward off type-2 diabetes-related health conditions, such as blood sugar control. When you eat according to the Mediterranean diet, it's obviously not a 100% guarantee that you'll never struggle with this disease; however, the odds look significantly more in your favor than when you're not on this particular diet.

6. Manages Pain Due to Arthritis

Rheumatoid arthritis is an autoimmune disease where the body's immune system attacks the joints. This creates swelling and pain in and around the joints. The Mediterranean diet is filled with anti-inflammatory omega-3 fatty acids, which greatly contribute to the pain management of arthritis. Of course, that doesn't mean that your diet should replace medication prescribed by a healthcare provider, but it can be an additional contribution to alleviating pain. Other diets, which aren't necessarily as rich in anti-inflammatory foods, won't have the same effect as the Mediterranean diet, so it's definitely the best course of action regarding food-specific treatment. If you struggle with joint pain or rheumatoid arthritis, the Mediterranean diet might be the best way to manage your pain and relieve some of the inflammation and swelling in your joints.

7. Fights Against Cancer

Various studies have found that the Mediterranean diet can help prevent certain types of cancer (Salomon & Lawler, 2022). More specifically, the Mediterranean diet can reduce the risk of breast cancer, colorectal cancer, and head and neck cancers. In cases where cancer has already been diagnosed, the Mediterranean diet can increase the chances of survival and prevent death (Salomon & Lawler, 2022). Women who are permanently on the Mediterranean diet have a 62% lower risk of breast cancer, which is extraordinary in itself! All in all, the Mediterranean diet is a great way of actively fighting off cancer and other life-threatening diseases.

8. Eases Depression

The last benefit I want to touch on is the finding that the Mediterranean diet can ease symptoms of depression. According to an analysis of 41 different studies, eating the Mediterranean way highly contributes to lower incidences of depression (Salomon & Lawler, 2022). In fact, when you're on the Mediterranean diet, you are 33% less likely to struggle with depression than those who typically follow a standard American diet that's filled with richer foods and processed meats

(Salomon & Lawler, 2022). Depression is a very dangerous illness that shouldn't be taken lightly, and anything that can help relieve the symptoms should be considered when you are struggling with depression.

These eight benefits are not just silly, minor benefits. These are highly beneficial elements to consider when you are evaluating the quality of your life. No wonder inhabitants in the blue zones live so long and happily! These benefits contribute to not only physical health but also emotional and mental well-being. The beauty of these benefits is that it doesn't require much from you. You have to eat, so you might as well eat according to the Mediterranean diet. It doesn't require you to do anything more than what you're going to do in the first place. So, let's be intentional with what we put into our bodies and start to take better care of ourselves in the long run. I hope you had the same reaction as I did as I worked through these benefits! I suddenly thought to myself, *Why wouldn't I eat the Mediterranean way when it's obviously so good for me?* Now that we know just how incredible this diet is, we can take a closer look at the Italians and the way that they implement this diet in their daily lives.

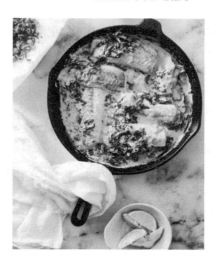

The Italian Twist

The Italians eat mostly according to the Mediterranean diet, but there are a few differences. Or rather, they put their own Italian twist on the already wonderful Mediterranean diet. With the goal of being as healthy as the Italians, we don't want to simply eat according to a new diet. So, what do Italians do differently? What is the Italian twist to the Mediterranean diet? Let's find out!

According to nutritionist Valentina Schiro, one of the best things about the Italian Mediterranean diet is that your plate will never be boring. Food is supposed to be enjoyed, not just tolerated. Since food and getting together to enjoy a meal is such a big part of Italian culture, it's cardinal that the food is delicious. People should want to get together and share food with one another (Altomare, 2019). There are three things that put the Italian Twist on the Mediterranean diet, which is what we'll look at next.

1. Veggies for Breakfast, Lunch, and Dinner

In an Italian-style Mediterranean diet, veggies are always the star of the show and should be added to every meal. They're not just the side dish or the add-on, but the protagonist that everyone loves. Well, for most of us, veggies might seem boring. How can you possibly have an interesting meal when you're adding vegetables to everything? Well, the secret lies in variation. Instead of having one or two vegetables that you have with every meal, experiment with different vegetables and the way that you cook them. Your plate should be a celebration of color with all the different vegetables!

This is often referred to as the "rainbow" plate. Your food shouldn't all be just one color. The more natural colors your plate consists of, the better. Different vegetables have different natural colors, which actually have different nutritional values. So, next time you're in the grocery store, be sure to not only add green vegetables to your cart but also other colored veggies, like eggplant, peppers, and pumpkin.

2. Yes, to Pasta

If you've ever traveled to Italy or watched a movie about Italy, you'll know that pasta is a big part of Italian culture. This contradicts many other diets that run from pasta as fast as they can. Even though the Mediterranean diet focuses more on vegetables and fruits, the Italian twist certainly prioritizes pasta. Most Italians eat pasta at least twice weekly (Altomare, 2019). Despite many diets painting pasta as the bad guy, that's actually not the case at all. Pasta is a complex carbohydrate that slowly releases energy in the body, and unlike most commercially available pasta, Italian pasta is made from whole grains that are locally sourced. This means that you'll have more energy during the day than when you eat other food or store-bought pasta. Pasta is also very digestible when combined with the right ingredients and consumed in quantity. Italians often mix their pasta with vegetables and a lot of tomatoes. Of course, they also add olive oil! When pasta and legumes are combined, they supply the body with essential amino acids, which contribute to muscle mass (Altomare, 2019). So, before you say "No, thanks!" to pasta, try making it the Italian way instead. Add vegetables instead of meat, and be sure to use olive oil when you're cooking.

3. Animal-Based Foods

While the Mediterranean diet doesn't completely restrict animal products, they are consumed less than in other diets. However, the Italians love their dairy products. They consume more cheese than others who follow the Mediterranean diet. However, they also eat very little red meat. Italians consume milk and dairy products daily and welcome fish and eggs as a source of protein several times a week. The meats they eat are mostly lean cuts, but they will eat almost any part of the animal. Red meat provides protein for muscle health, and organ meats are one of the most nutrient-dense foods available. Italians aren't known as vegans, although some do follow a vegetarian diet. Animal products are highly appreciated in the Mediterranean diet and are considered the best source of protein and nutrients. Even though Italians consume more cheese than others on the Mediterranean diet, they also consume cheese within limits. They also don't add cheese to every meal but rather use it as an appetizer or with olive oil and bread. While in the States, many foods are covered in cheese, the Italians have a more subtle approach. Quality over quantity is certainly one of their mottos when it comes to cheese consumption.

Despite these three differences that the Italian twist adds to the Mediterranean diet, there is also a different approach to seasoning food than the rest of the world. As mentioned, olive oil is used liberally for dressing. Herbs and aromatic plants are also found as a part of nearly every recipe. Italians season food liberally with basil, parsley, rosemary, oregano, and bay leaves. Italians definitely don't stick to the salt-and-pepper basics, and they also don't season their food by adding more fat and calories as heavy sauces.

This brings us to the end of this chapter. I hope that you now have a better picture of what the Mediterranean diet looks like and how the Italians put their own twist on the diet. But there's more to how Italians eat than just what they eat. Italians have a distinct food culture that is uniquely different than other parts of the world, and that is exactly what we'll look at in the next chapter. If you take away only one thing from this chapter, remember that pasta isn't the enemy, despite what other diets might suggest. Are you ready to learn more about Italian food culture? Let's get right to it!

Chapter 4
The Italian Food Culture

Mangiare per vivere e non vivere per mangiare—Eat to live, don't live to eat.

When a reporter asked Giorgio Locatelli, an Italian chef, what it means to have an Italian lifestyle, he said that there are two things that you should think about as soon as you open your eyes in the morning: what you are going to have for lunch, and what you look like (Lorne Blyth, 2016). The food culture in Italy goes beyond just simple nourishment, it's about so much more than just feeding your body. In fact, they believe that the way you cook speaks volumes about your personality. Chef Locatelli mentioned how his family heavily distrusted their neighbors because they added parsley to their minestrone. How you cook your food is one of the most discussed topics in Italy and amongst locals, with very little consensus. This is due to locals being deeply proud of their Italian food culture, and they certainly wouldn't take it lightly if someone were to offend their cooking style.

Much of the food culture in Italy is deeply rooted in a rich history, which we'll get to in this chapter.

That's not all that we'll be discussing. We'll also look at the diversity in Italian food (Be warned, not everything is about pasta and pizza). We'll look at two very rich food cultures in Italy: the coffee culture and the wine culture. Finally, we'll end this chapter by looking at ways that we can incorporate the Italian food culture into our own lives, no matter where in the world we find ourselves. Before we get to that, I want you to take a moment and think about your own food culture. It's easy to look at other food cultures and think, *That's so strange!* but we all have some food cultures that make us different. In America, there is a big food culture following the "the bigger, the better" method. We want to make the biggest hamburgers, the largest milkshakes, and a record-breaking barbeque. This is something that other cultures find extremely strange and is even considered wasteful.

Soon after my wife and I got married, I made a big mistake: I compared her cooking to my mother's cooking. I lovingly mentioned how my mom would make lasagna, which was my absolute favorite. It goes without saying that my wife made it her life's mission to make the *very best* lasagna. While she made lasagna exactly how her mother and grandmother did, it was... good but different to me. We both had our own family food cultures that subtly clashed with one another. Well, it's the same in Italy, with every family, region, and village having their own twist on the food culture. However, there are a few things that remain the same. Those are the ones we'll focus on, but first, let's explore the history of Italian food.

History of Italian Food

While in many countries we don't really give two thoughts about the history of our food, in Italy, it's quite the opposite. Not only to the generational history within their dishes, but the history of Italian food, as we know it today, dates all the way back to ancestral Rome. Of course, it has evolved and transformed over the years, but the root of Italian food still goes back to Roman traditions of kings and warriors (Bezzone, 2019). The love for food in Italian culture started at the Roman banquettes, a place where new dishes were tried, and the empire embraced new flavors. They started incorporating different flavors and spices from the other lands that they conquered, especially from the Middle East and the shores of the Mediterranean. The Romans developed a taste for fine cuisine with intricate flavors prepared with sophisticated techniques. However, this was only how the wealthy lived. The general public used what was referred to as the Mediterranean triad: bread, olive oil, and wine (Bezzone, 2019).

This expensive and sophisticated style of feasting quickly came to an end when Rome was conquered by "Barbarians," and the empire collapsed. The Central and Northern European conquerors had very little in common with the Romans, and their lifestyles and different cuisines influenced one another. They brought butter and beer to the common household, while the Romans taught them the use of olive oil and a taste for wine (Bezzone, 2019). During the middle ages, things changed dramatically. After Sicily became an Arabic colony, spices, and dried fruits became a common concoction. It was also the Arabs who brought dried pasta to Sicily due to its long shelf life. From Sicily, dried pasta was transported to Naples and Genoa and quickly reached every nook and cranny of Italy. Along with pasta came religion as well. Christianity came to Italy with many rules on how to live and what to eat, which significantly influenced the Italian diet. Specifically, Italians started eating less and less meat while implementing fasting periods.

The Conquerors and the Christians had opposite diets, but the two were reconciled by Charlemagne, who declared some days as fasting for all, followed by heavy feasts. Both sides started incorporating these rules and enjoyed good food more than ever (Bezzone, 2019). In the later middle ages, something new took root in the Italian towns: community culture. Communities began building strong relationships with their neighbors and started sharing products with ease, paving the way for merchants. The economy was doing much better thanks to the merchants, and food once again became a symbol of enjoyment and class. Sugar cane was introduced by Arabic influence, and this changed the culinary game, as the kitchens started experimenting with sugar instead of honey (Bezzone, 2019). Arabs also introduced lemons and oranges to Sicily, and most importantly, marzipan. The cassata, which is the most popular Sicilian dessert, was also created due to Arabic influences. One of the best-kept secrets is the world-famous Italian dessert, gelato, which was also influenced by Arabic tradition.

As we can see, the history of Italian food has many different influences, which all evolved into a very rich Italian culture filled with food and dessert that are celebrated across the globe. Even though much of the praise should go to the Middle Eastern influences, Italians eventually put their own spin on the recipes, which is the Italian food we know today. Although pizza and pasta are what Italian food is best known for in the world today, Italian food is far more than just pizza and pasta. Different regions in Italy are actually renowned for diverse and unique cuisines. In the next section, we'll find out more about the diversity of Italian food.

The Diversity of Italian Food

To say that Italians are only known for their pasta and pizza is like saying Elvis was only known for his dancing: It's simply not accurate, and it's almost insulting. There are many things that contribute to the diversity of Italian food, but the two most obvious influences are the change in times and the historical influence on the different regions. Northern Italy started developing dishes based on meat and butter, thanks to Northern and Central European influences, while Southern Italy focused on fish-based dishes and different types of cheese. There is also much diversity when it comes to bread and pasta. In the Northern regions, Italians started exploring with fresh pasta, which led to ravioli and tortellini, while the South explored with dry pasta (Capatti & Montanari, 2016). The city of Milan was the birthplace of risotto, while Bologna made tortellini. Florence gave us the famous Fiorentina, and Napoli created pizza as we know it.

Of course, climate and natural landscape also play a big role in the different cuisines. In Alba and the surrounding areas, expensive truffle mushrooms are well-known and loved due to their natural growth there. However, when you're in Tuscany, you are more likely to enjoy a beef steak, thanks to the cattle raised in the Chianina Valley (*Exploring Italian Cuisine*, 2019). Even the cheeses in different regions vary. In Campania, you'll find soft cheeses, while in Sardinia, you'll find harder and saltier cheeses. The Italian regions take a lot of pride in their creations, which is why you'll often find that products are named after the region that they're created in. For example, Modena balsamic vinegar can only be crafted in Modena, and Parmigiano Reggiano cheese is only produced in the provinces of Emilia-Romagna. Bread also varies in different regions. Italian bread differs in size, taste, and texture. Ciabatta loaves are from Lombardy's Lake Como, while in Turin, you'll find crunchy breadsticks instead (*Exploring Italian Cuisine*, 2019).

While Italian cooks can argue for hours about the proper way to prepare certain dishes, there are also numerous similarities in the way that they serve and enjoy their meals. Instead of serving everything in one big meal, Italians serve food in an array of small plates that are enjoyed in succession. This is what makes meals so special in the culture: Italians take time to savor the different meals. The appetizer, or as it's called in Italy, the antipasto, is served first, followed by a course of pasta or other starches. Then, meat or fish with vegetables is served, followed by salad, cheese, fruit, and coffee (*Exploring Italian Cuisine*, 2019). While in other countries, dessert is served after the main course, in Italy, dessert is often enjoyed as a midday snack along with coffee.

The diversity in Italian dishes is what makes it so special. While every region has its own specialty and twists on things, they all agree that meals are more than just about food, but about coming together and enjoying each other's company. This is something that we can most definitely incorporate in our own lives to ensure longevity and health.

The Coffee Culture

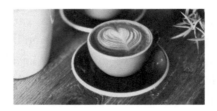

Coffee culture is a big thing not only in Italy but around the world. A quick stop at your favorite Starbucks isn't a strange concept for most of us, and drinking coffee to wake up in the morning is a pretty normal occurrence in most households. However, the Italians have a slightly different approach to coffee than the rest of us. For Italians, coffee isn't just something that you have, it's a culture that you join and enjoy. Interestingly enough, Italy doesn't grow its own coffee beans. In most places in Italy, the climate and the terrain simply aren't suitable for coffee farms. Traditionally, Italian coffee grounds are Arabic. However, during the Second World War, Italy struggled to import beans from Arabia and started getting their coffee from Northern Africa. The Arabica coffee is a smoother and more acidic flavor, while the Robusta coffee (found in Northern Africa) is thick-bodied and stronger flavored. So, if Italy doesn't even grow its own beans, why is Italian coffee such a big deal? Well, it's all about the preparation.

Generally speaking, Italian coffee is a darker roast than what we're used to. Italians also drink it slightly differently than the rest of the world. While we're used to standing in line at Starbucks, looking at a long list of different coffees with flavors available, Italians keep it a little bit less fluffy. Here's a list of eight types of coffee that you can find in Italy:

1. **Caffè**: The most common coffee in Italy is an espresso. Usually served in a small cup, this is the go-to for most Italians. They often enjoy a quick espresso during the day with a pastry of some sort (Dombrowski, 2015). When you go to someone's house and are offered coffee, this is most likely what you'll get. Espressos are strong, served without milk, and usually drunk quickly. It serves as a quick pick-me-up and helps with some extra energy and motivation.

2. **Cappuccino:** This is another favorite in Italy. However, if you order a "grande" or a "venti,"

Italians will raise their eyes and think to themselves, "Another American!". A cappuccino is a cappuccino, and there are no different sizes. In Italian, venti literally means "20", so if you order a venti, you might just end up with 20 cups of cappuccino! A cappuccino is ⅓ espresso, ¼ steamed milk, and ⅓ foam (Dombrowski, 2015). If you're not quite accustomed to the strong taste of an espresso, a cappuccino is a safer bet for you when visiting Italy.

3. **Macchiato**: A macchiato is the perfect combination of an espresso and a cappuccino. Served in a small cup, like an espresso, this drink packs a punch but isn't as strong as an espresso. A macchiato consists of an espresso with a touch of drops of hot froth. It's not as frothy or milky as a cappuccino, and it's also enjoyed throughout the day (Dombrowski, 2015).

4. **Marocchino**: This is the beautiful creation of coffee combined with chocolate. While it's not a chocolate coffee in the sense of it being flavored or added together in a blender, it's rather built in the mug, like art. It starts with a shot of espresso, followed by a layer of foam, and on top, you'll find cacao powder. Unlike the other coffee, the marocchino is served in a glass mug that has been dusted with cocoa powder. It's milkier than a macchiato, and the cocoa gives it a stronger but sweeter taste. In some regions of Italy, they add a layer of thick hot chocolate before adding the foam layer (Dombrowski, 2015).

5. **Caffè Latte:** If you order a tall latte in Italy as you would in the States, you will end up with a

glass of milk. What we call a latte is actually a caffè latte, which means coffee and milk. A caffè latte is served in a taller glass mug and consists of ⅓ espresso and ⅔ heated milk, with a little bit of foam on top. Since this is so milky, Italians only drink this before 11 a.m. and not in the afternoons. If you're not a fan of strong coffee, a caffè latte is the perfect solution for you.

6. **Shakerato:** What we call an iced coffee, Italy calls a shakerato. Often served in a cocktail glass, like a margarita, the shakerato consists of an espresso poured over ice, and then shaken to a froth. No milk is added, unlike most iced coffees that we know. A shakerato is often enjoyed in the mornings during the summer since the other option for something cool (Aperol spritz) is only acceptable after 11 a.m.

7. **Caffè al Ginseng:** Have you ever had a chai tea latte? It's quite popular in the US and in other countries, but quite impossible to find in Italy. The closest to a chai tea that you'll find is a caffè al ginseng. This delicious coffee consists of espresso prepared with ginseng extract and no other sweeteners since ginseng is naturally quite sweet. This is a great energy booster and also aids in digestion. It's often enjoyed after meals to help with digestion and to boost you for the rest of the day. Also served in a small espresso mug with no milk, this is another strong coffee that you finish with a couple of sips.

8. **Caffè d'Orzo:** This is Italy's version of a decaf coffee. A caffè d'orzo is 100% natural and a great way to include the kids in coffee culture. It's often

served with a slice of orange to give it an extra fruity taste. Many Italians enjoy this drink late at night to avoid feeling too buzzed to fall asleep.

Italian coffee culture is quite proud of its coffee creations, and many Italians can be quite stubborn when it comes to their drink of choice. If you try to give them something else, they might simply refuse to drink it, especially if it's something with seven consecutive names that includes whipped cream and sprinkles on top. They probably won't even acknowledge that as coffee. Well, that might just be the key to their coffee culture and why it's actually good for their health. Since most Italian coffees have very little sweetener and almost no milk, it's healthier than how we consume coffee in other countries. There are many benefits to drinking coffee the way that Italians do. These benefits include:

- protects against heart disease
- lowers the risk of a stroke
- reduces the risk of developing type-2 diabetes
- protects against Alzheimer's disease
- reduces the risk of gallstones
- promotes regular digestion
- reduces the risk of cancer
- helps with fat burning
- aids in dental health
- prevents headaches

No wonder coffee culture is such a hit in Italy and that Italians live the healthiest lives on earth! Well, before we move on to the next section, grab yourself an espresso and get ready to explore Italy's wine culture.

The Wine Culture

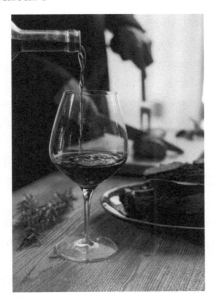

Italy has a very rich wine culture that is rooted deep within its history. Even before the Roman Empire was a thing, Italians enjoyed wine. Before Rome, the Greeks revered the god *Dionysus*, who later became the god of wine and pleasure, who the Romans called *Bacchus* (Bartalesi, 2023). Even though Italians enjoyed wine before the Greeks arrived, the Greeks introduced them to new wine-making techniques, allowing the wine culture to truly flourish. When the Greeks studied the vines and cultivars in Sicily upon their arrival, they were so impressed that they called Italy, Land Oenotria, which means "the land of trained vines" (Bartalesi, 2023). During these times, wine was made by foot stomping and was fermented in terracotta storage jars. It was an incredibly popular drink since it was safer to consume than their polluted water. During the reign of the Roman Empire, the wine market grew even more. The Romans believed that wine was a necessity, so it was available to all: women, slaves, and aristocrats. Pompeii was one of the biggest wine regions of the time, which caused a spike in wine pricing after the volcanic eruption that destroyed the vineyards (*The History of Wine*, 2021).

In the 19th century, Italy's wine quality began to diminish. To prevent this from happening even more, the government began regulating the industry with a series of labels. The different labels were used to tell the public that the winemakers met the specific requirements and that the wine was of good quality. To this day, Italy uses these labels (*The History of Wine*, 2021). They are:

- Denomination of Controlled and Guaranteed Origin (DOCG). This is the highest degree of quality.
- Denomination of Controlled Origin (DOC)
- Typical Geographical Indication (IGT). This is the broadest category.
- Quality Wine Produced in Specified Regions (VQPRD)
- Table Wine (VDT)

Italy is the leading wine producer, producing 19% of the world's wine. So, it's safe to say that wine is a big deal in Italy. Italian winemaking follows a simple, five-step process (*The History of Wine*, 2021):

1. **Harvest**: All the best wines begin with an excellent harvest. In Italy, they harvest grapes in the winter. The grapes are kept in open containers, which they call gondolas. While some farms harvest grapes by machines, others still believe in harvesting by hand.

2. **Crushing**: Once the grapes are ready, the stems are removed, and they begin the crushing process. They are moved to the crusher, where the grapes are pressed to produce juice.

3. **Fermentation**: After crushing, the berries are sent to fermentation. They are put into vats where they start the fermentation process. Some grapes are fermented in small oak barrels to add more flavor and aroma. Yeast is also added to the barrels to begin fermentation.

4. **Aging**: Before the wine gets bottled, they are left to age. The duration of the aging depends on the type of grape, but it's usually between 6 and 24 months.

5. **Bottling**: Finally, the wine gets bottled, and they remove all the impurities. Depending on the wine and the wineries, they either make use of natural corks or screw caps.

One of the biggest things to note about Italian wine is the importance of the region. Each region has its own specific qualities, and they are very proud of their own wine. The rain, soil conditions, and quality of the sun all influence the type of grape they harvest and the taste they acquire. There are a few regions in Italy that stand out above the rest as the wine regions (*The History of Wine*, 2021).

- Veneto
- Piedmont
- Lazio
- Sicily
- Umbria

- Tuscany
- Sardinia

The average Italian consumes one bottle of wine per week since they enjoy wine with every meal. The wine culture in Italy contributes to their health since we know that wine in moderation has a lot of health benefits. No wonder the Italians live so long and happily! Wine is also an incredibly powerful antioxidant that prevents cell damage. Antioxidants can also prevent many diseases, such as heart disease and certain cancers. Yes, that's right! Wine might just save your life, literally! However, take note from the Italians and keep wine drinking in moderation; otherwise, it would do the exact opposite for your health.

Incorporating the Food Culture

The question of how we can start incorporating the Italian lifestyle is yet to be answered. We know that Italians highly value the history of their food and honor the regions where certain meals originated, but how can we incorporate their way of living from across the globe? Well, we can use what we've learned so far on this journey and focus on the way that they approach food instead of simply trying to copy and paste everything that they do. Perhaps we can leave out the superstitions, like believing that spilling olive oil will bring bad luck, and keep the principles that make them such a healthy country. Here are seven habits that we can learn from an Italian food culture that we can incorporate into our daily lives (Bensalhia, 2016).

1. Keep Breakfast Light and Simple

While many people believe that your breakfast should be big, hearty, and filled with all kinds of meats, eggs, and bread, the Italians believe quite the opposite. Breakfast in Italy is quite a modest affair. You won't see plates filled with fried food and bacon. Instead, they keep breakfast light and easy. It usually consists of coffee, bread rolls, or cookies. In the smaller areas of Italy, other popular choices for breakfast consist of fruit salad, yogurt, and muesli (Bensalhia, 2016). Some Italians don't have breakfast at all but enjoy a snack around 11 a.m. The reason why most Italians eat a light breakfast is because they are saving their appetite for their biggest meal of the day, which is lunch.

2. Keep it Fresh Because Fresh Is Best

Most Italians make use of local markets and shops to get their groceries instead of larger-scale supermarkets. They also value growing their own produce, especially in the smaller villages. Italians value fresh food and would very rarely buy frozen vegetables or meat. They believe in making everything from scratch and making it fresh. Due to busy schedules, we often tend to gravitate toward frozen or pre-made food that we can just quickly pop in the oven. However, when food gets frozen, it loses much of its nutritional value and flavor. For most Italians, cooking is an art, not just something they must do. That's Italians believe that getting it fresh is best! We can start to incorporate this in our lives by looking for local markets or simply using fresh products to cook instead of frozen foods. Sure, it might mean a few more trips to the grocery store, but for the added flavor and health benefits, it's worth it!

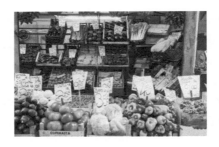

3. Veggies Daily, All Year Long

Speaking of fresh produce, after a closer look at the Mediterranean diet, it's safe to assume that we all know just how important vegetables are for Italians. However, what many of us don't realize is that they only use vegetables that are in season. While we find vegetables in the supermarket all year round due to importing and genetically modified foods, Italians focus on eating what is naturally in season. During the summer, they eat a eggplants, beans, beetroot, cucumbers, zucchini, peas, and tomatoes (Bensalhia, 2016). However, when the winter months arrive, you'll find artichokes, broccoli, Brussels sprouts, cabbages, cauliflowers, and spinach on their tables. Vegetables that grow all year round, like chicory and carrots, are enjoyed throughout the year. We can start incorporating this habit by becoming aware of what vegetables are in season and when and looking for markets where we know the produce is fresh and not imported.

4. Heavenly Gelato

Another thing that Italians enjoy during the summer months is gelato. Gelato is a healthier alternative to ice cream since it contains less sugar and is made from a slower churning process. Gelato is also known to include fresh fruits that are frozen to create a natural sweetness. In the southern parts of

Italy, they enjoy sorbet, which doesn't use any milk, but only water. So, next time you're craving a sweet treat, opt for a gelato or a sorbet instead of creamy, sugar-filled ice cream. It's still delicious and will most definitely scratch the itch for something sweet and cool! On a warm day in Italy, you'll find a gelato stand on every corner and in everyone's hand, so join the club and get yourself some gelato.

5. Simple Suppers

Since lunch is the biggest meal of the day for Italians, Italians keep their suppers simple and on the smaller side. Not only are their dinner small, but they also tend to be simpler and less extravagant than lunches. Many of the meals that Italians enjoy at dinner originated among peasants during the Roman Empire era. They often eat soup and bread for supper, especially during the colder months of the year, and naturally enjoy flatbreads and pizzas the rest of the year. Dinners often consist of leftovers that are slightly jazzed up to create a delicious new dish. Many of us, on the other hand, eat our largest meals at night and usually eat something fairly simple and small for lunch (Bensalhia, 2016). Large meals at night don't allow the food to be fully digested before bed. We can start incorporating this habit by focusing on smaller dinners and keeping them on the simpler side. This will also give more time to relax in the evenings instead of spending a lot of time cooking.

6. Pizza!

Speaking of pizza, the Margherita pizza is a big fan favorite in Italy, and many Italians eat pizza on a daily basis. For them, it's more like bread than an elaborate process with loads of toppings on it. The fact is that originally, pizzas were only a round base with no toppings at all (Bensalhia, 2016). In the 18th century, it became very popular due to its inexpensive ingredients but still being delicious. The Italian Queen, Margherita of Savoy, wanted to taste what pizza was like. Despite raising eyebrows in the court circle, she asked the chef, Rafaelle Esposito, to make her a pizza. He agreed but made it slightly fancier than how the commoners ate it. He added tomato and mozzarella cheese, along with fresh basil. He used the ingredients to represent the red, white, and green colors of the Italian flag (Bensalhia, 2016). It quickly became the Queen's favorite, so the tradition of the Margherita pizza was born. We can incorporate the habit of a simpler pizza by opting for a delicious Margherita pizza instead of one with many toppings and complicated pronunciation. Take it back to the root of it all and keep it simple and delicious!

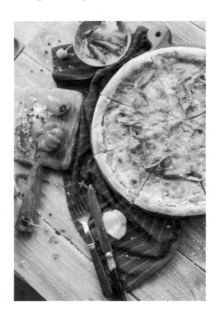

7. Tomato Sauce

The first thing that most diets tell you to cut out is sauces. It's a well-known fact that sauces can be quite fattening and are usually filled with sugar to give them a nice taste and to help with the preservation. However, there's one sauce that is actually relatively healthy, especially if we make it the Italian way. That is, of course, tomato sauce! Tomatoes have numerous health benefits and can even prevent certain diseases and chronic illnesses. We can incorporate this Italian food culture by swapping our other sauces with simple tomato sauce, prepared the Italian way. Many Italians make their own tomato sauce at home to ensure it's fresh and filled with preferred spices.

Of course, we can also incorporate the coffee and wine culture of the Italians by ensuring that we drink our coffee as they do and by enjoying wine in moderation. By implementing these habits, we're well on our way to living the Italian way, at least when it comes to food. However, there's more to the Italian food culture than just what they eat. The Italians also make use of something called "The Slow Food Movement," which is what we'll look at in the next chapter. First, take some time and think about three Italian food culture habits that you can start to incorporate today.

Chapter 5
The Slow Food Movement

Va piano, va sano, e va lontano–Go slow, go healthy, and go far.

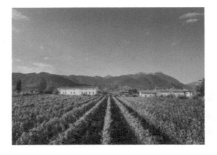

Recently, I was speaking with a colleague who mentioned his wife had just called and asked him to pick up dinner - again. Last night the Golden Arches, the night before pizza. He marveled that my wife always prepared a home-cooked meal for our family. He said his wife just couldn't do that because she is in no mood to cook after a long day of stressful clients and even more stressful management meetings. Besides - he said - she doesn't enjoy cooking because the kids are so spoiled they won't eat anything but hamburgers and fries, mac and cheese, or pizza. *Goodness*, I thought to myself, *that's a life of fast food!* His family isn't unique. It is estimated that one out of three Americans eats fast food on any given day, especially those aged 20-39 and 34% of children. (Shari Mason, 2023). The market size of the quick service restaurant (QSR) industry in the United States was 322.05 billion U.S. dollars in 2021, up from the previous year's total of 301.49 billion U.S. dollars. In 2022, the market size was forecast to reach 331.41 billion. (Statistica). As I drove home, I started thinking about these astounding numbers and the quality of all of that fast food. It's so common for people to call a delivery service or stop for take-out, despite knowing that fast food isn't the healthiest. It's become so normal that we don't really give it much thought.

The following day, I was still wondering about this whole "fast food" concept when I stumbled upon a blog in my junk mail titled *Join The Slow Food Movement*. I honestly had no idea what it meant to be part of a slow food movement, so I decided to do some research and read up on its meaning. To my surprise, it was a very Italian way of doing life. Not only a healthier way of life but also a healthier approach to caring for the earth. Sounds a little bit too good to be true, right? Well, it doesn't come easy, especially not in a culture where we try to do everything as quickly as possible, including eating and preparing food. However, it is possible, and Italians have done it for decades. This chapter will explore the slow food movement and everything that comes with it. We'll look at the history of the slow food movement and what it means. We will also look at slow food movement habits that we can incorporate to live longer, happier lives.

Are you ready to dive into the world of slow food movement? Trust me - you won't regret it!

The History of the Slow Food Movement

The slow food movement originated in Italy in 1989 and was founded by Carlo Petrini. He wanted to promote traditional preparation methods and a way of life that came with pleasure, peace, and a love for food. Petrini believes that food has the power to bring people together and unite communities with their environment (*Slow Food Movement Guide*, 2021). With fast food, you don't really think about the food you're eating or the impact that it might have on the environment. You place your order, pay, and eat. Slow food, on the other hand, focuses on being conscious and mindful of what you're eating, how it's prepared, and how it impacts the environment. The goal is to respect seasonality, reduce environmental impact, and support local producers and culinary traditions (*Slow Food Movement Guide*, 2021).

The idea of the slow food movement started when Petrini noticed that the connection between the farmer and the consumer had been severed due to capitalism and large supermarkets. He noticed that there was no longer a true sense of respect toward the earth, and few people knew where their food was coming from. Petrini says that the movement was born out of two events that took place. The first was the opening of a McDonald's restaurant in the Piazza di Spagna in the center of Rome. He strongly believed it diminished the Italian way of cooking and eating. The second event was when cheap wine was sold to locals, which led to the death of 19 people. The wine was made with methanol and poisoned thousands of people (*Slow Food Movement Guide*, 2021). He realized a profound loss of heritage was taking place and that people had to reconnect to their Italian roots and way of living.

Although the slow food movement is still very unknown outside of Italy, many Italians have converted back to their traditional way of eating and understanding Italy's food origins. So, what exactly does the slow food movement represent, and how can we join the movement and implement these elements into our homes? I'm glad you asked! Let's discover what the slow food movement believes before we consider how to incorporate these habits into our lives.

The Slow Food Movement Beliefs

The slow food movement envisions a world where people can access and enjoy food that is inherently good for them and good for the planet (*Our Philosophy*, 2015). The slow food movement believes in three interconnected principles:

- good
- clean
- fair

These three principles formulate their manifesto, and it is their pledge to work toward a better future. According to the slow food movement, when we live interconnected with these three principles, we will unlock a tool to help improve the food system we are accustomed to today (*Our Philosophy*, 2015). The movement wants to connect the farmer and the consumer once more to create unity and care for the planet. However, whether you're the producer or the consumer, you can play a role in the slow food movement and work toward a better, healthier future with a sustainable planet. These three principles are ultimately at the core of everything they do, so let's take a closer look and try to understand what they represent.

1. Good

The slow food movement doesn't want to take away the goodness of food that you're enjoying. Actually, it's quite the opposite. They want to reconnect with the goodness of natural food that is filled with flavor and aroma. Unfortunately, if you have untrained senses, you are more likely to miss these aromas and flavors, which is why they want to educate the consumer to reconnect with the products and the goodness (*Our Philosophy*, 2015). They believe in keeping food's goodness by avoiding alteration or preservation. The more natural the food, the better it will taste. Good food is a big part of Italian culture and is essential for health and wellness.

They clarified this principle when they first protested the rise of fast-food restaurants in Italy. Instead of simply handing out flyers and making signs, they handed out bowls of freshly cooked pasta to everyone who passed them. They didn't want to take away food from people but rather reconnect people with quality, flavorful, and healthy food. They made it clear that they didn't want fast food; they wanted slow food.

2. Clean

The second principle of the slow food movement revolves around clean eating. Now, clean eating doesn't mean what it means to most people who are on a diet. Clean eating has more to do with the environment and how we should respect the world we live in. The goal of the slow food movement is to practice farming, processing, marketing, consumption, and animal husbandry in a way that is sustainable and respectful to nature (*Our Philosophy*, 2015). Every stage in the agro-industrial production chain plays a part in the well-being of the environment, even if you're just a consumer, and every stage should take into consideration how their behavior is affecting the earth.

That's why every stage should try to protect the ecosystem and not just exploit it (*Our Philosophy*, 2015). When you practice clean production and consumption, you are safeguarding the health of the consumer as well as the producer. The slower the food process, the healthier the outcome. When we try to modify certain natural processes to perform faster, we ultimately choose wealth over health.

The slow food movement encourages production that isn't harmful to the environment, which is why they market to local producers instead of corporately owned supermarkets (*Our Philosophy*, 2015). They believe that every person should start their own garden and support local farmers instead of buying into mass production.

3. Fair

The third principle that the slow food movement believes in is fairness. They believe that social justice should be pursued by creating conditions that respect people's rights (*Our Philosophy*, 2015). Producers should be rewarded fairly for their farming, and costs should be reduced by removing the middleman, which is the distribution chain. At the moment, farmers don't receive enough compensation, while consumers have to pay increasingly larger amounts for food. Why? Because the middleman is calling the shots. The slow food movement wants to achieve a balanced global economy through the practice of solidarity and sympathy. They also believe in respecting cultural diversities and traditions, which should be celebrated. Large corporately owned supermarkets force smaller markets to conform, removing the special traditions that each of them has (*Our Philosophy*, 2015).

The slow food movement wants to bring fairness back into

the spotlight by granting accessible prices for the consumer and fair conditions for the producers.

Above and beyond these three principles, the slow food movement believes that the work should be implemented locally, nationally, and internationally. In 2018, a study found that seemingly similar food products bought in supermarkets could have two very different influences on the environment. The problem is that the consumer isn't aware of this and often chooses the cheapest options. This ultimately comes down to a lack of clear labeling. Furthermore, the study found that food production creates 30% of the world's greenhouse gas emissions, not to mention the amount of food waste that most families throw away on average (*Slow Food Movement Guide*, 2021). Due to all these factors, the environment, consumers, and producers are drawing the short straw and suffering greatly.

You and I might not have a large effect on the international state of things, but we can certainly influence our local market and decide how we want to spend our money, but that's not the only way that we can incorporate a slow food movement into our daily lives.

Slow Food Habits

It might be daunting thinking about concepts of change for the greater good, but this change is also good for your own health and longevity. In Italy, the idea of slow food has taken deep root and is becoming more and more popular again. Just think back on the blue zones and how most of them made their own food from scratch and shared mealtimes with others, taking enough time actually to enjoy it. So, why can't we embrace it in our own homes? It may not be the easiest way, but it certainly is the healthiest and most beneficial way of enjoying food. Here are a few ways that you can incorporate the slow food movement at home (*Change Your Habits*, 2022).

- Research the labels of products that you buy off the shelf, and don't consume anything with more than five ingredients.
- Don't eat anything as a meal that your grandparents wouldn't consider food.
- Don't eat anything that contains ingredients that you can't understand or pronounce.
- Only consume food that will eventually rot and doesn't last forever.
- Do eat fermented food that bacteria or fungi have transformed.
- Avoid supermarkets when you can and opt for local markets.
- Start your own garden.
- View meat as something you consume on special occasions and not something that needs to be on your plate daily.
- Eat animals that were fed well and were considered healthy.
- Look for signs on the label that say the product is part of the Fair Trade and is organic.
- Research brands to ensure that they are ethical.
- Reduce your carbon footprint by only consuming food that is in season.
- Plan meals in advance and only buy the ingredients that you'll use.
- Use fresh ingredients to cook and not frozen foods.

We can all do our part to embrace the slow food movement. Not only is it good for you and your family, but it's also good for the earth and for future generations. Take a moment to identify three ways that you can start incorporating slow food into your daily lives. In the next chapter, we'll explore another part of Italian culture that contributes to longevity and health: family and tradition. As soon as you've identified ways to incorporate slow food into your schedule, you're ready for the next chapter. I'll see you there!

Chapter 6
The Importance of Family and Traditions

A tavola non si invecchia—At the table, you don't get old.

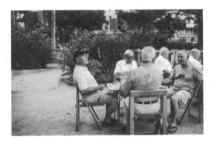

I talians never eat alone. That's not me guessing or assuming; it's true! They don't eat alone unless they really can't help it. Italians always share a meal with family and friends, and of course, that includes *Nonna* and *Nonno* (grandparents). There's something special about sharing a meal with friends and family. I must admit, we used to enjoy meals together as a family when the kids were younger, but as they grew older and time passed, and our work schedules filled up, it became less of an everyday thing and more of a once-a-week thing. I never really noticed how much it affected us until one Sunday when we all had time to spend together.

It wasn't any Sunday, but a beautiful Easter Sunday, and we had a magnificent home-cooked meal planned. The kids were all home or in town, and everything was perfect. The meal was to die for - an antipasto of cheese, salumi, and homemade bread, a first course of gnocchi made with ricotta, eggs, and organic flour, with a light sauce of tomatoes and basil, a main dish of roasted lamb cooked with garlic and rosemary, along with broccoli di rapa in garlic and olive oil and an arugula salad. We had an amazing time! We laughed and caught up on how everyone was doing. It felt almost like a movie moment. You know, those feel-good Hallmark movies where there's always a happy ending? That's how it felt. I leaned back in my chair and watched as everyone was listening to one another, enjoying each other's company, and for the first time that week, I didn't have a headache.

When I started reading up on how Italians spend their days, it made complete sense to me why Italians value eating with family and friends so much; I thought back to that spring day and realized just how special it was. Imagine if we shared times like this not just on holidays but every day! No wonder they live so long and happily! Community and companionship are more important than we think. In this chapter, we'll look at the benefits of having a strong family bond and how eating with your family can contribute to that healthy bond. We'll also examine Italian family roles and how the dynamic works within their families. Lastly, we'll look at Italian traditions that keep them connected and how they celebrate these connections together. I want to encourage you to keep an open mind as we go through these points and write down when you have an idea of how you and your family and friends can spend more time together. Allow yourself to dream a little and buy into the idea of spending more time with the family.

Benefits of a Strong Family Bond

I know that spending time with family isn't always all roses and sunshine. Most families fight with one another or sometimes just annoy each other endlessly. However, at the end of the day, they remain family. Being part of a family is a gift; if you live near your family, it's an even greater gift! However, it can get a little sticky when your brother annoys you or your father-in-law wants to tell you how to use your barbecue. That's why it's so important that we focus on the good side of the family and spend quality time together to cultivate those relationships. Spending time with family is incredibly important in Italian culture, and for good reason! It's not just because they actually enjoy each other's company, but it's also because spending time with those you love can be highly mentally and physically beneficial for your health. Let's have a look at the eight benefits of spending time with family and friends.

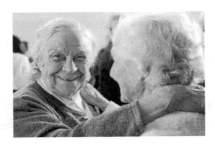

1. Stress Relief

My children are seriously funny. I know most parents laugh at their kids or think that their jokes are the best, but I can confidently say that mine make me laugh until I cry!

Whenever I have a bad day, I call one of them and spend a few minutes talking. I immediately feel better, especially if they're in a silly mood. No wonder I feel so much less stressed when they're home for the holidays or come to visit us. Family ties have been shown to provide stress relief for individuals, and they can greatly help family members get a fresh perspective on the issues and challenges they're facing (Meleen, 2021). According to research, having a strong family bond can prevent troubling feelings since family acts as a shield, protecting from negative emotions and troubles. People with strong family ties are more resilient and tend to have better coping mechanisms when faced with stressful situations (Meleen, 2021). Italians spend a lot of time with their family and friends. It provides a sense of security. Knowing that you belong is probably one of the greatest confidence boosters for an individual, and it highly contributes to overall happiness and inner peace. Can you think of a moment when spending time with family helped you to forget about stressors in your life?

2. Healthier Diets

When you sit down to enjoy a meal together as a family, it tends to be a healthier meal than what you would have had when you're alone. For so many friends, whenever their "family cook" is away, they rely on takeout or snacks to keep them full. Instead of cooking up a storm just for themselves, they eat chips while lying on the couch. However, when the chef returns home, the entire family comes back together. Across all ages, when family members eat together as a unit, they tend to be healthier (Meleen, 2021). Usually, family meals mean less processed food and more vegetables. Since family ties are so important in Italy, they ensure that everyone is included in the cooking process and meals. While grandparents may skip meals when they're alone, when they live with the family and take part in the cooking, they are more likely to eat healthy meals. When you spend time with your family, you might still get takeout occasionally, but in general, you'll eat meals that are balanced and filled with nutritious value. When you compare the meals you have when you're alone to the meals you have when you're with family, how do they compare?

1. Regulates Emotions

According to studies, when you spend a lot of time with your family, you are more equipped to regulate your emotions in a healthy manner (Meleen, 2021). Children who spend a lot of time in the presence of other family members show better emotional control and regulation than those who don't spend time with family. The more time you spend with your family, the more you'll be held accountable when you're behaving in a way that's not considered appropriate. This teaches you how to act, making you more self-aware. With better self-awareness comes the ability to know what you're feeling and to deal with it appropriately (Meleen, 2021). Italians are passionate people, but they tend to be good at regulating their emotions. When you spend time with your family on a daily basis, you need to learn how to control your emotions in a healthy way; otherwise, you might get called out for it. The family also creates a safe space for you to express your feelings and be heard. Your family should be your sounding board, which helps you make sense of everything that goes on outside the family dynamic. Do you think spending time with your family will help you regulate your emotions better?

2. Longevity

This is no surprise since longevity seems to be a theme that constantly pops up when we look at Italian culture. Well, the more time you spend with family, the better your chances of living a long and fulfilled life. In a long-term study, researchers found that individuals without family members are twice as likely to die young than individuals with strong family relationships (Meleen, 2021). The study also found that the stronger family connections you have, the better your chance of living a long life. When you are connected to your family, you feel supported and happy in a way that no other person can make you feel. That's why it's so important to have family support when you're going through a difficult time or when you're recovering after surgery. When you have family who loves you and who is waiting to help you, you are more likely to survive traumatic events (Meleen, 2021). Since Italians live longer than most of us, we can surmise family plays a big part in it. Do you have family members that can help you through difficult times and be your source of recovery when you go through a traumatic experience?

3. Prevents Crime

Spending time with family members can reduce crime in society. I know this sounds too good to be true, but you best believe it! The reason is that people who spend time with family exemplify the overwhelming benefits of family versus the behavior of those who don't. A recent study looked at prisoners whose family members came to visit them often, and it found that prisoners who receive family visits are 40% less likely to become repeat offenders than those who never receive family visits. When you have a family, you change your behavior accordingly, even when you've made a bad decision. Having someone to support you and love you even when you make a mistake aids in your behavior, leading to a lower risk of behavioral problems. This can also be seen in children with an active family bond and those without. Children with absent parents are more likely to cause problems and get into trouble than children with a steady family bond. You might not prevent crime in the sense of changing other people's behavior but in the sense of ensuring that your family stays out of trouble. Can you think of a time that your family kept you from doing something slightly stupid that would have gotten you into trouble?

4. Economic Prosperity

Not only is it an emotional benefit to have a close family, but it can actually lead to economic prosperity (Meleen, 2021). A recent study showed that people who naturally spend a lot of time together become the major economic contributors to society (Meleen, 2021). This is because bigger and closer families sharing similar values also mean that there are more contributing adults who generate an income under one roof. Since Italians spend a lot of time with family, they cook together and even help around the house, so they don't spend money on cleaners or daycares to look after the children. Children usually stay with their grandparents or great-grandparents if both parents work. If you have a tight-knit family, you will also contribute to each other's wealth in how you live and help each other accomplish various goals (Meleen, 2021). In what way has your family contributed to your economic prosperity?

5. Improves Mental Health

Spending time with family also means that you are more likely to have good mental health (Thatcher, 2020). The first way to battle mental illness is often by spending more time with those you love. When you have depression and anxiety, you might want to isolate yourself, which only worsens the symptoms. However, when you spend quality time face-to-face with your family, anxiety is reduced, along with depression and any other symptoms that might come with it (Thatcher, 2020). Being physically present with the ones you love creates a strong emotional support system that helps you face life's obstacles with courage. Italians have a lot of resilience and do not struggle with mental health, especially in the smaller villages. A big part of that is thanks to their quality family time with their family and friends. Can you think of a moment when your family really helped you through a dark time and improved your mental health?

6. Teaches Conflict Resolution

The last benefit of spending quality time with family that I want to highlight is the fact that it teaches how to resolve conflict. When you spend a lot of time with family, you'll probably also fight with them more and more. However, unlike other relationships, with family, you don't get to walk away and ignore the issue! Especially if you're seeing them again the next day. Instead, it teaches you to express your feelings and talk things through. It also teaches how to say sorry and how to forgive others (Thatcher, 2020). Spending time with family teaches interpersonal communication skills that include healthy ways to discuss problems and how to debate without hurting the other person. Italians are very passionate people, but they quickly forgive and move on from past issues. They don't hold a grudge but believe in forgiving each other quickly. How has spending time with your family improved your conflict resolution?

Looking at these benefits, it's clear that having a family you spend a lot of time with is wonderful. If you don't have a big family or aren't in contact with your family, don't worry. That doesn't mean that you can't reap these benefits. It simply means that you have to be intentional with creating a family bond with your friends. A family isn't always just through blood; it can also be through choice. The Italian family culture and their friendships are extremely important to them. Now that we've discussed Italian family culture, we also need to discuss Italian family structure.

Italian Family Structure

Family life in Italy is often described as loyal and filled with close ties. The family structure is larger than what most other cultures are used to. They don't just consider the nuclear family as "family," but also all extended relatives. Family for Italians stretches over several generations, and they are often the foundation of a certain neighborhood or village (Thomas, 2022). Italians have a much stronger feeling toward family than they have toward their country. Their families are the most important aspects of their lives, and when they move to new areas or even countries, they often take their extended family members with them. Extended families often live together, and in most Italian homes, the grandparents take an active role in childcare (Thomas, 2022).

- **Children**

Children are watched over carefully, and from a very young age, they are trained to be loyal and obedient to their elders. Italians believe that every member of the family should have a role, so children often get tasked with chores and errands from a very young age. It's incredibly important to Italians that children respect their parents and other elders in the community, and children are often expected to give up their seats when elders walk into the room (Thomas, 2022). While it's becoming more and more common to have only two or three children, the family still plays a big role in the upbringing of the children. Children are also taught from a young age not to embarrass their family name and to uphold a good reputation.

- **Gender Roles**

Italian women are known to be strong and independent. That's not by accident! In fact, women are encouraged to be bold from a very young age, making them renowned for their confidence. Despite independent women, Italy has quite a traditional approach to gender roles. Catcalling and whistling is very common behavior when you see a beautiful woman, and women are often stereotyped as beautiful but unintelligent. This makes it slightly harder for women to pursue a serious career and often face lower wages. Even though men and women have equal rights by law, Italian society is still largely male-dominant (Evason, 2017). The man is usually the primary income earner and the leader of the house, while many women are stay-at-home mothers. Even when women have jobs, they are responsible for taking care of the household responsibilities.

- **Dating and Marriage**

Couples in Italy often get engaged very young but wait until the man has a stable job before getting married. Engagements are often a couple of years without a set marriage date. Marriage is a respected covenant in Italian society, and celebrations are often held in the bride's hometown. The bride and the groom are not allowed to see each other the day before the wedding, and families also prefer that their children marry other Italians. Italians are only allowed to get a divorce after being legally separated for six months (Evason, 2017). Living together before getting married isn't a strange concept to Italians since the average age for marriage is between 27 and 30. In general, the regions in the south of Italy are still more traditional than the northern regions of Italy.

Other than the family structure, it's also important for us to look at Italian traditions since it plays such a big role in how they live together as a community.

Italian Traditions

Italy is rich with traditions that are passed down through many generations. It's not uncommon to find a craftsman in Italy that learned the skill from their great-grandfather and who is planning on teaching his own child one day. Italians take incredible pride in their craft, and they work hard to become masters in food, architecture, design, furniture, fashion, and painting (Prentice, 2020). The smaller towns in Italy are especially rich with wonderful art and crafts. Let's have a look at three examples of how Italian craft has been passed down to the next generations.

1. Cinabro Carrettieri

On a small hilltop located in the Val di Noto region in Sicily, you'll find the small town of Ragusa. In Ragusa, you'll find many Italians keeping the Sicilian folklore alive in the way that they craft different carts. These carts were used by businessmen to transport goods and played a big part in Sicilian culture. One of these crafters is a painter who has spent his entire life painting Sicilian carts. He paints old stories of historical literature and religions on these carts, stories that were told to him as a child. The Sicilian artists also use their ancient craft on modern-day furniture. One painter, in particular, collaborated with Dolce & Gabbana to create a Smeg kitchen appliance collection representing the Sicilian art of cart making (Prentice, 2020).

2. Nicola Fasano Ceramics

In the southern region of Puglia, you'll find the small town of Grottaglie. Grottaglie is widely known for its ceramics and the incredible ceramic experts who live there. Franco Fasano is one of the great ceramic heads who reside in Grottaglie, which doesn't surprise anyone! The art of ceramics has been in the Fasano family for 18 generations, and they have special family techniques that they only share with their family members. They produce all their ceramics in-house, and buyers can choose from a great variety of ceramic art. Nicola Fasano became especially popular with his splatter-print tableware and is known to push his design style further with every new collection (Prentice, 2020). Nicola has worked with some big names in the industry and recently collaborated with Giorgio Armani.

3. Arte Ferrigno

Italy is a very religious country, so when it's Christmas season, the streets of Via San Gregorio Armeno in Naples are filled with people looking for nativity shops. This street is known for all its different nativity shops, especially Marco Ferrigno. The nativity artisanship has been in his family since 1836, and he recalls spending hours as a child watching and learning as the others created the special art pieces. Thanks to Marco's excellent training, he has gained some popularity internationally and has made figurines of some of the world's most famous celebrities. He makes all of his figures by hand and spends his hours carefully crafting the different emotions he experiences.

These are only three examples of how Italian traditions often transfer from generation to generation. This also creates a bonding moment for the family as everyone spends their time together, learning the different crafts. Take a moment and think about your own life. What tradition can you carry on or pass down to your family? In the next chapter, we'll look at the Italian lifestyle and how they manage to stay fit without any diet.

Chapter 7
The Italian Lifestyle

Non potremmo avere una vita perfetta senza amici—We cannot have a perfect life without friends.

You remember that meeting I told you about earlier where I experienced the slow food movement for the first time? Well, I didn't only experience the slow food movement during my travels to Italy. In fact, I discovered that many Italians live according to *Lo struscio*, which means "slow living." Instead of being trapped in a hustle culture, like most are, the Italians have a more peaceful approach to life which undoubtedly contributes to their longevity and overall health. It's hard to comprehend slow living when you're used to running around, chasing deadlines, and trying to get everything done before midnight. I found it strange at first, watching as people strolled down the street, taking time to chat to one another, and even greeting strangers. However, the more I thought about it, the more I realized that perhaps we were strange and not them.

When was the last time you did anything slowly? Personally, my life has been a bit like a runaway train since college. I constantly chased the next achievement, trying my best to stay on track with everyone around me. Perhaps you feel the same way? It almost seems impossible to do anything slowly because then you'll fall behind the rest. Well, imagine if everyone just stopped rushing. Wouldn't that be glorious? Well, that's exactly what Italians do. Don't get me wrong, they still work hard and have goals, but they also take time to smell the flowers and create deeper connections with others. This is what they call slow living. It's all about being in the present and enjoying the life you have. What's the point of rushing when you never feel like you've made it anywhere? The slow living approach to life aids in mental health as well as physical health. Not to mention, it's also so much better for your relationships with others!

In this chapter, we'll look at the different areas of a slow lifestyle. We'll look at how friendships play a big role in Italian culture and health and how we can build friendships that last. We'll also explore the Italian work culture and look at the biggest differences between them and the rest of the world. Finally, we'll look at how the slow-living culture contributes to maintaining a healthy weight and why it doesn't make you gain weight like most people fear it would. Embracing the different aspects of slow living can help you live a life you enjoy and contribute to your overall well-being. So, be open-minded and ready to embrace a new way of doing life.

Friendships in Italy

Having friendships are incredibly important during all ages of your life. However, we often overlook the importance of friends as we get older. We never really look at a woman in her 90s and ask her who's her best friend, but perhaps we should start! Italians have a very special approach to friendships. They believe that friendships begin during infancy and that it lasts a lifetime (Thomas, 2022). Dante, the father of Italian literature, believed that living a perfect life without friends is impossible. Many friendships in Italy reach far beyond just one specific season; they endure a lifetime. Even in big cities, friendships are highly valued, and it would be strange not to introduce yourself to your neighbors.

Friendships in Italy are also less planned. You would very rarely make plans weeks in advance but would rather be impulsive and show up unannounced at someone's home with a bottle of wine and dinner. In Italy, friends also often meet up by accident. When you run into a friend, you naturally spend the rest of the day together. You don't say "hi," and then quickly rush off. While friendships are considered important all over the world, it's often overlooked in the older ages. However, in Italy, Italians believe that growing old with friends is even more important than growing old with a spouse. They also believe that your friends keep you young, and you would often see a group of elderly people out on the town doing something that they love.

Italy almost views friendships as the family that you choose. Friends share everything with one another, including hardships and celebrations. You can see this after a new baby is born. It's almost as if the whole town starts celebrating! Research has shown that friendships are essential for seniors, and not just because it's fun, but because of the many health benefits. Let's have a look at six reasons why friendship is essential during all ages of your life (8 *Reasons*, 2023).

1. Physical Health

Many studies have shown that people with good friend-ships maintain better physical health, especially as they age. A strong sense of friendship makes you less likely to suffer from heart disease, high blood pressure, and obesity. Just think about little kids running around the playground. The person with many friends is usually the person who is the most active and the person who is constantly being called to join the game. The one without friends is often the one who sits in the corner, not moving. The same goes for seniors. Seniors with friends are more likely to go for a walk together or enjoy gardening. They tend to be more active, which boosts their physical health (8 *Reasons*, 2023).

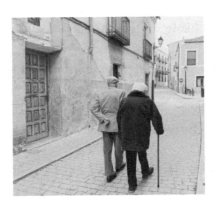

2. Loneliness and Isolation

Feeling isolated makes you more likely to struggle with depression, dementia, and other disabilities. Isolation can be very dangerous, especially with age. Many people assume that older people don't mind being alone, but the opposite is actually true. It's essential that older people find like-minded friends with whom they can talk to. Whether to chat about their children or about a new hobby they've picked up, it's important for them to have companionship to fight feeling lonely. Italians understand this concept of friendship, so they make friends not only for a specific season but also for life.

3. Cognitive Health

As strange as it might sound, when you have friends, you are less likely to experience cognitive problems when you get older. Friends offer care and support, which contributes to feeling less stressed. When you live a life that's not over-whelmed with stress, you will have more gray matter in your brain as you get older, which prevents cognitive problems (*8 Reasons*, 2023). A study done in recent years found that 60-year-old people who only saw friends every couple of months were 12% more likely to develop dementia (*8 Reasons*, 2023). That's partly why Italians spend so much time with friends throughout their lives. Older generations still form part of the community with an active role.

4. Better Self-Esteem

When you have friends, you feel like you belong and like you are part of a group. Having friends gives you a purpose, especially as you age. Research has found that older people with friends have better self-esteem than those without (*8 Reasons*, 2023). When you have friends, you are likelier to partake in activities that boost your happiness, like joining a community or volunteering. That's why the Italian elderly are known for their ability to be active within the community and for having good self-esteem (*8 Reasons*, 2023). The stronger your social network, the more enhanced your personal development will be.

5. Through Thick and Thin

Friendships are precious in the sense that they last through many seasons. When you have friends that stay with you through thick and thin, you are more likely to recover after a traumatic experience. For example, if you have good friends, you are more likely to be okay after the death of a spouse than if you were completely alone (8 *Reasons*, 2023). We can look to the Italians to witness this firsthand. When something happens to someone in the community, everyone comes together and helps those around them.

6. Better Behavior

The last benefit of having good friends that I want to point out is the fact that friends encourage healthy behavior. Of course, we're all responsible for our own lives, but good friends encourage each other to be healthy. In Italy, many elderly citizens encourage each other to go for long walks or to visit the market together. Friends encourage each other to be active and mobile, which contributes to overall health (8 *Reasons*, 2023). It's important to have friends that encourage healthy behavior, and equally, so should you also encourage healthy behavior in your friends.

Having friends that last a lifetime is essential if you want to live a full and happy life. That doesn't mean that you can't make friends when you move or when you're not in touch with those you went to preschool with anymore. Rather, it acts as a reminder to be intentional with friendships wherever we go, just like the Italians. Despite having such an incredible friendship culture, Italians also have a different work culture than most of us are used to, so let's look.

Work Culture

Italy is known as a country with a good work-life balance. No matter your career choice, you are expected to prioritize your family and rest often to ensure that you remain healthy and contribute to the success of the organization. The maximum work hours per week is 40; if you work overtime, it can't exceed 48 hours (Bolla, 2020). Many organizations close for a midday *riposo,* which means an afternoon rest. Organizations that honor the *riposo* will typically close between 1 p.m. and 3:30 p.m. Italians work 36 hours a week and receive four weeks of paid holiday on average. They also have access to 12 public holidays and strict labor contracts to ensure that all workers maintain a healthy work-life balance (Bolla, 2020).

Of course, how much you work also depends on your sector. Especially in the bigger cities, the private sector can expect to work longer hours. Most private sectors work from 9 a.m. to 6 p.m. with an hour lunch break. Public offices, on the other hand, work from 8 a.m. to 2 p.m. Even night workers aren't allowed to work longer than 8 hours within a 24-hour shift. Italians highly value their summer holidays, and many organizations close during the month of August to enjoy a summer break (Bolla, 2020).

In Italy, they also approach work with a more casual style. They have good relationships with their employers and focus on maintaining modern, casual conditions within the work-space. Some companies allow workers to choose their work hours based on availability. Many companies also make use of 6-month contracts to ensure that workers have the ability to leave if they wish to do so (Bolla, 2020). Meetings are often conducted over extended lunch breaks where good food is shared.

Maternity leave is also much different in Italy than in the States. Female employees aren't allowed to work during the two months prior to the planned delivery, and new moms are entitled to 80% of their salary during maternity leave. Mothers are sometimes allowed additional time off when they have dangerous or physical jobs. Italians highly value recognition within their industry and often get rewarded with monetary prizes, verbal praise, written tributes, or financial bonuses (*Characteristics of Work Culture in Italy*, 2022). In Italian work culture, hierarchy is highly respected, and companies tend to have a pyramid-shaped hierarchy. While open communication and feedback are welcomed, the boss always has the ultimate say, even when they work in a more relaxed environment. General ambiance and friendliness are highly valued, and colleague conflict is very rare.

Speaking of colleagues, in Italy, getting to know those you work with is very important, which often happens over a 90-minute lunch break. Bonding is a key part of the team, and it's essential that you make friends with your colleagues to avoid getting too stressed at work. Colleagues often go for a walk over lunch breaks or enjoy each other's company while sharing a meal. Having these positive relationships at work can help you manage stress and feel more at home (*Characteristics of Work Culture in Italy*, 2022). Colleagues also keep you accountable and often send each other home if they work too much overtime.

With all of this being said, how can we incorporate this into our daily lives? Well, if you're an employer, you can make sure that your work culture values personal and professional lives. If you're an employee, you can start by being friendly to your colleagues and by having boundaries to ensure you get enough family time. In short, Italian work culture includes:

- shorter workdays
- flexible hours
- comfortable and casual relationships
- respect
- lunch breaks
- a lot of vacation days
- honoring public holidays
- rewards beyond salary

This healthy work-life balance culture highly contributes to Italians' overall health and productivity. Despite what many might think, many studies have found that people who work shorter days are more productive than those with long hours. It also contributes to physical and mental health, which we should all strive for.

How Italians Maintain a Healthy Weight

Speaking of good physical health, you'll find very few over-weight citizens when you visit Italy. Many people find this surprising since they assume that Italians live on pasta and bread. However, Italians actually maintain a very healthy diet, as we've seen, and they also focus on staying active. In fact, they actually have a name for this. They call it *passeggiata*, which refers to a short walk taken purely for pleasure (Ludwig, 2017). Many Italians take a *passeggiata* multiple times daily, most commonly after a meal. When you're in Italy, you'll barely notice the difference. People don't wear spandex and giant water bottles with them while "exercising" because they're simply walking for the pure enjoyment of it (Ludwig, 2017).

This enjoyable walk is the quiet secret to why Italians remain so slim. Many researchers have found that taking a short walk after a meal can highly contribute to weight loss, and it can even decrease the risk of developing diabetes. These short walks are often more helpful than one long exercise, and you also reap many other benefits besides weight loss. A short walk after every meal will actually aid in digestion, and it also aids in your sleep hygiene. The best part is that it doesn't even feel like exercising.

Italians tend to go for a walk instead of watching television late at night after dinner. In that way, they also spend time with the people they love and build relationships. It's the best of both worlds. You and I can start incorporating this method right away. Instead of spending your evening on the couch, take a 15-minute walk and see how you feel afterward. This might just be the stress reliever that you need! Other than the *passeggiata*, Italians have another secret that aids in their health. They call it *Dolce far niente*, which means "The art of doing nothing."

While many of us dread the feeling of doing nothing and often chase the next thing on the list, Italians enjoy the sweet feeling of doing nothing and being idle. This isn't because they're lazy but because they value rest and peace. They use this term to describe leisurely relaxation (Brittney, 2022). Put simply, they enjoy doing nothing. For Italians, it's not a waste of time to relax or spend weekends resting. Even when meeting up with friends, they will schedule a time to do nothing and rest both physically and mentally. The art of doing nothing is often hard to achieve, especially in modern work culture and thanks to the fear of missing out (FOMO). Many people are so scared that they'll miss out on something that they fear sitting still.

The concept of doing nothing is rooted in Italian history, which we can see in the art where people are lounging around or relaxing in hammocks. It's all based on the notion that happiness can be found in the small moments and in the little things, like taking a break (Russell, 2019). Italians make time to do nothing while drinking coffee or eating some gelato. Italians often use this time to laugh at tourists or even politicians! They find things to laugh about around every corner and take time actually to listen to jokes (Russell, 2019). While many seek relaxation by traveling or buying something we don't need, Italians have learned the art of relaxing by doing nothing. Instead of saving up to go someplace far, Italians use their money to enjoy life as it is now.

So, how can we enjoy the art of doing nothing? Well, we can start by doing the following things:

- Take a random day off from work and don't do anything. Don't tell anyone you're taking the day off (except for your boss), and don't fill it with plans or chores. Do nothing and enjoy doing it.
- Use your free moments in your daily routine to do nothing. Instead of checking emails or packing out the dishwasher, take a moment to do nothing.
- Mean it when you say you want to do nothing. Log out of social media, put away your phone, and do nothing that connects you to the outside world.
- Take a nap and enjoy the fact that you can take a nap without feeling guilty. The work will still be there when you wake up, so just take a nap and experience the bliss.
- Enjoy a glass of wine just because. Don't wait for a special moment or for someone to visit. Enjoy a glass of wine and simply sit with the nothingness.

We can all start enjoying the sweet art of doing nothing as a way to relax and rest. In this chapter, we've learned that there are many things about the Italian family culture, work culture, and rest culture that we can implement into our daily lives to be healthier and happier. Next, we'll take it a little further by looking at some of the best Italian recipes you can try at home this week. As we're nearing the end of this journey, we can start to implement the things we've learned so far and continue on the path of health and longevity.

Chapter 8
Healthy Italian Recipes to Try at Home

Troppe salse vivande false—Too much sauce means false food.

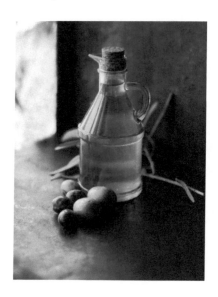

I t's time to start cooking and eating like an Italian. If you have no idea where to start, don't worry. We'll face this together! Even if you're not a MasterChef, these easy Italian recipes will fill your kitchen with delicious aromas in no time! All you have to do is choose a recipe, read it through, get the ingredients, and follow the steps. These recipes are all fairly easy to get you up and running the Italian way without spending endless hours cooking. Of course, use your own imagination and creativity with the recipes. If you want to add an additional ingredient, go for it! Feel free to customize the recipes to cater to your specific needs. If you find a recipe that you like, why not invite the family over for a lunch party this weekend? Let's do life the Italian way without holding back! Happy cooking!

Sardinian Herb Soup

Italians love making soup, and in winter, you won't find an Italian home without a pot of some sort of soup on the stove. One of the most popular soup recipes in Italy comes from Sardinia. Herb soup is quite popular all over Italy, and every region and family adds their own twist to it. This specific recipe focuses on the herbs of Sardinia and delicious Italian cheese. This soup is often called S'*erbuzzu*, and it consists mainly of different green vegetables, beans, meat, and pasta. Originally, this soup was made with all the herbs and vegetables that grew naturally on the island of Sardinia. This soup is fresh and filled with herby goodness.

Time

- 40 minutes

Serving size

- Four servings

Notes

- You will use the parsley's stems and leaves but separate them during the preparation since they'll be used during different phases.

Ingredients

- Two tablespoons of extra virgin olive oil
- kosher salt and black pepper grounds
- Three large, minced garlic cloves
- 1 ½ teaspoons of fennel seeds
- Two quarts of chicken broth
- ¾ cup pasta of choice (fregola is recommended)
- Four ounces of diced pancetta (use bacon if you can't find pancetta)
- One bunch of parsley
- Four ounces of baby arugula leaves.
- ½ cup fresh chopped tarragon
- ½ cup of dry white wine of your choice
- Fifteen ounces of white beans (fresh or canned)
- Two ounces of hard cheese like Romano (grated)

Directions

1. Start by prepping the ingredients. You can grate the cheese, set it to the side, and separate the parsley

stems from the leaves. Cut the arugula and tarragon into rough pieces.

2. In a pot, heat your olive oil and cook your meat. Let it cook for about 6 minutes, and then add the parsley stems, the fennel seeds, your wine of choice, and some grounded black pepper.

3. On medium heat, let the mixture simmer for about 3 minutes. This will allow most of the liquid to evaporate.

4. Add the chicken broth to the mixture and let it boil. Once it boils, lower the heat, and add the pasta. Allow it to simmer for about 10 minutes.

5. After 10 minutes, add the garlic, parsley, the white beans, and some of the cheese. Let it simmer for another 10 minutes.

6. Remove the soup from the heat before adding the tarragon and arugula. Add some salt and pepper to your liking.

7. Add a little bit of cheese on top and serve warm.

This soup also makes for great leftovers! So, if it's a family favorite like I expect it to be, make a large pot and keep some for the next day as well.

Sardinian Tomato Salad

Usually, when people read the word "salad," they skip over the page to the following recipes. Well, I highly suggest you stick around for this salad! It is filled with Sardinian goodness which holds the key to longevity. Sardinian salads are often different in each household, with everyone adding their own flavor to it, so don't be afraid to explore with some added ingredients yourself. This salad is filled with tomatoes, rocket, and other green goodness. Enjoy!

Time

- 40 minutes

Serving size

- 6–8 portions, depending on how hungry you are

Notes

- You can use whatever tomatoes you like best! Try to find tomatoes that are currently in season, and be careful not to use unripe, green tomatoes since they are best used when you want to pickle tomatoes. I recommend using cherry tomatoes since they are nice and sweet.

Ingredients

- sea salt for serving
- salt and pepper for seasoning
- One clove of garlic, not chopped but only halved.
- ¼ cup of extra virgin olive oil
- Two tablespoons of vinegar of your choice
- ½ teaspoon of orange zest, freshly grated
- Two tablespoons of fresh orange juice
- One loaf of ciabatta bread
- 2 ½ pounds of fresh tomatoes cut into wedges
- One bulb of fennel
- ½ cup of green olives, pitted

- One tablespoon of fresh parsley
- One handful of fresh rocket (arugula) leaves.

Directions

1. Start by prepping the ingredients. Chop the parsley and slice the fennel into thin pieces. Cut the tomatoes into smaller pieces and squeeze your orange to get some juice. Place your onion in a small bowl of iced water and let it stand for at least 10 minutes.
2. Whisk together your orange juice, zest, and vinegar of choice. Add the olive oil and some salt and pepper.
3. Add tomatoes, fennel, dried onions, and olives in a different bowl. Add the vinaigrette that you made in Step 2. Allow the salad to stand for at least 15 minutes or longer. It can stand up to 2 hours and still be fresh, so if you want to make it in advance, you are more than welcome!
4. Just before serving, add the parsley and some more salt and pepper. Remove the salad from the mixing bowl and add it to a serving plate. Drain the juices into a pitcher and use as a salad dressing.
5. Toast your ciabatta and rub it with olive oil and garlic. Sprinkle your salad with salt, pepper, and fennel.
6. Serve the tomato salad with the bread and some additional salad dressing.

You can eat this as a main course or serve it as a side dish to another meal. Feel free to add other ingredients like cucumber and green bell peppers.

Insalata di Tonno e Fagioli

In simple English, it's a tuna salad. But who wants to call it a tuna salad if you can call it *insalata di tonno e fagioli*? Regardless of the fancy name, this salad is super easy to make and so delicious! Of course, it's even better when you use fresh ingredients, but if you can't find any, it also works with canned beans and tuna. This dish is usually served as an antipasto right before a bigger meal, so if you're making it as your main meal, add some more ingredients to prepare a bigger salad.

Time

- 30 minutes

Serving size

- Serves four people as an antipasto

Notes

- If you're using canned tuna, look for tuna in olive oil, not those in brine. This will enhance the taste and make it healthier. Prep your cannellini beans a couple of hours before serving the salad.

Ingredients

- One onion chopped thinly
- One tablespoon of extra virgin olive oil
- Salt and pepper to taste
- Two tuna steaks or canned tuna
- 14 oz cannellini beans

- One handful of parsley

Directions

1. You can prep your cannellini beans the night before since they need time to soak. Place your beans in a container and cover them with clean water. Let them soak for a couple of hours or overnight. Then, bring the beans to a boil on high heat. Remove the beans from the heat and scoop off the foam on top. Bring to a boil again and allow it to boil for 10 minutes. Let it drain and cool down before adding the beans to the salad.
2. Chop your parsley roughly and prep your other ingredients accordingly.
3. Salt your onion and cover it in cold water. Leave it for about 10 minutes, then remove it from the water.
4. Add the olive oil to a pan and fry your tuna steaks with some salt and pepper.
5. Mix the onion, parsley, and beans. Flake your tuna and add it to the salad mixture. Season with more salt, pepper, and olive oil.

You can also serve this salad with a vinaigrette sauce or with balsamic vinegar.

Walnut Pesto

This meal, quite literally, tastes like something you'll find in a fancy restaurant in Italy. However, it's so easy to make! You can choose whether you want to serve this pesto with a side salad as a main dish or whether you want to serve it as an antipasto. I recommend using zoodles (which are zucchini noodles), but you can also use spaghetti if you prefer that. However, the zoodles option is healthier and slightly better for your longevity.

Time

- 20 minutes

Serving size

- Serves six people

Notes

- This recipe pairs beautifully with some red wine, so go full Italian and pour yourself a glass.

Ingredients

- Two tablespoons of kosher salt
- ½ cup extra virgin olive oil
- 6 quarts of water
- Two large garlic cloves that you've minced
- 1 cup cherry tomatoes
- 1 cup grated parmesan
- 2 cups of chopped spinach
- One tablespoon of chopped parsley
- Three zucchinis for the zoodles or 1 pound of spaghetti
- ¾ cup of walnuts

Directions

1. Start by prepping your walnuts and placing them in a food processor for a couple of seconds. Stop as soon as the walnuts form a crumbly texture.
2. Peel your zucchinis to make zoodles. If you're using spaghetti, cook it until it is al dente.
3. In a large pan, add your nuts, garlic, parsley, and olive oil. Cook it on low heat for 5 minutes or until the mixture turns golden brown. Don't use high heat since that will cause your walnuts to burn.
4. Add your cherry tomatoes, diced spinach, and zoodles to the pan. Cook until everything is golden brown. If the sauce is too thick, add ½ cup of water.
5. Serve with parmesan on top and some extra fresh parsley.

Enjoy the meal, and remember the glass of wine! It's easy, delicious, and perfect to share with family and friends.

Italian Minestrone

I can honestly say that this is probably my favorite meal of all time! Nothing warms the heart quite like an Italian Minestrone. This dish is incredibly satisfying and is filled with veggies, noodles, and delicious flavors. It's perfect for any occasion, and you can decide how simple or elaborate you want to make it. A minestrone is perfect when you have a couple of random ingredients in your house and are unsure what to make with it. You can either make this meal in a standard pot on the stove or use a slow cooker and let it cook on its own.

Time

- 40 minutes

Serving size

- Serves 8 to 10 people

Notes

- You can easily make this recipe gluten-free by using gluten-free noodles.
- If you have other vegetables in the pantry that are not listed in this recipe, feel free to add them to the mix! This was traditionally made from all the leftovers, so don't be scared to experiment with different kinds of vegetables.

Ingredients

- Seven tablespoons of extra virgin olive oil
- One onion, chopped into smaller pieces
- Two garlic cloves minced
- Two celery stalks, chopped into smaller pieces
- 28 ounces of crushed tomatoes
- ⅓ cup of chickpeas
- 1 cup of beans of choice
- Two carrots, chopped (peeling optional)
- Three potatoes, diced (peeling optional)
- 2 cups chopped fennel
- ½ cup Italian parsley leaves
- 1 cup pasta of choice
- fresh basil leaves
- salt and pepper

Directions

1. Start by prepping all the ingredients and cutting all the vegetables into smaller pieces.
2. Add the olive oil, onions, and garlic into a pan and cook until brown. Add the carrots and the celery and cook for 5 minutes.
3. Add the crushed tomatoes, potatoes, herbs, beans, chickpeas, and other vegetables to the mixture. Let it simmer for 20 minutes. When the potatoes are soft, you can remove the pot from the heat.
4. Add the dried pasta to your mixture, add back to the heat, and cook for 10 minutes.
5. Season the minestrone with salt and pepper and add the fresh basil leaves on top right before serving.
6. Dig in and enjoy!

This recipe is sure to be a family favorite, so be sure that you make enough that there are also leftovers.

Eggplant Parmesan

This eggplant parmesan is an incredibly comforting dish, and it's so easy to make. It's also healthy and low in calories, so you don't have to feel guilty when indulging in this delicious meal. Even if you're not an eggplant fan, this recipe will make you change your mind! I've seen little kids who hate veggies ask for seconds, and even teenagers eat with a smile. Enjoy!

Time

- 60–70 minutes

Serving size

- Serves six people

Notes

- The tomato sauce is an essential part of this recipe, so be sure to use a quality sauce. I recommend adding some basil and garlic to the tomato sauce to enhance the flavor. If you want something with a bit of a bite, add some chili flakes or red pepper.

Ingredients

- extra virgin olive oil for cooking and drizzling
- 1 cup of shredded mozzarella
- 1 cup of parmesan
- Two garlic cloves
- 24 ounces of tomato sauce
- pepper and salt
- Two eggplants, cut into slices
- 1 cup of breadcrumbs
- Two eggs (3 if they are on the smaller side)
- basil and rosemary for seasoning
- Two tablespoons of water

Directions

1. Start by preparing the ingredients. You can grate the cheese in advance and dice and slice all the needed veggies.
2. Preheat your oven to 400°F and coat a baking dish with olive oil.

3. Mix your water and eggs together. Then, in a separate bowl, mix your breadcrumbs, parmesan, and seasoning together.
4. Dip your eggplant slices into the egg mixture, then coat it with the breadcrumb and cheese mixture.
5. Place the eggplants on a baking tray and add some more olive oil. Bake the eggplants for 30 minutes, flipping them over halfway through. Season with salt and pepper when they come out of the oven.
6. While the eggplant is baking, you can mix your tomato sauce, garlic, basil, and crushed pepper together.
7. Spread the tomato mixture in the oven dish and layer the eggplant slices on top of it. Add more sauce and then follow with cheese. Repeat the layers until you reach the top of the dish or until the ingredients are finished. Top with the remaining cheese.
8. Bake for another 20 to 30 minutes, then let it cool for 5 minutes before serving it with fresh basil and white wine.

You can also add other vegetables like mushrooms and squash if you have that in the pantry. This is sure to be another family favorite recipe to enjoy together!

Zucchini Frittata

A frittata is a flat omelet you can fill with whatever vegetables you have, and of course, with some cheese. This dish is healthy and so easy to make. It's a great impromptu brunch recipe, or you can serve it as a main course with a side salad. If you want to exchange the ingredients in this recipe for something else, you are more than welcome to!

Time

- 35 minutes

Serving size

- Serves two people

Notes

- This gluten-free recipe is a meal to make when you have friends or family over with gluten intolerance. It's also vegetarian, even though meat lovers can choose to add cooked ham.

Ingredients

- 4 teaspoons of extra virgin olive oil
- ½ cup of onion, chopped
- ½ cup of cherry tomatoes
- 1 cup zucchini, diced
- ¼ cup of fresh mint
- ¼ cup basil
- salt and pepper for seasoning
- Five large eggs
- Two ounces of feta cheese

Directions

1. Add the olive oil to a skillet and warm it up. Add the onions and cook until it is brown. Add the zucchini and cook for a couple of minutes, until tender.
2. Add the tomatoes, mint, basil, salt, and pepper to the mixture and stir over medium heat for a couple of minutes.
3. Beat the eggs and some salt together. Add the zucchini mixture to the eggs and add the cheese.
4. In a clean pan, add a little oil and the frittata mixture. Don't stir the mixture; leave it for 2 to 4 minutes. Once the top is golden and the egg starts to lift on the side, remove it from the heat.
5. Cut it into slices and serve.

If you want to add meat, add some diced ham or bacon to the frittata mixture before adding it to the pan. You can also garnish the frittata with fresh basil, mint, or a couple of tomatoes.

These recipes are only the beginning. I highly recommend investing in a Mediterranean diet cookbook or a blue zone recipe book. Experiment with different flavors, and remember, cooking is an art. You get to be creative! So, add whatever you think would be delicious and put your own twist on these Italian dishes. Whether you're a beginner in the kitchen or an expert, these recipes will be perfect for you. Implementing what you've learned on this journey is all up to you, so start with what you're putting into your body. Besides, the meals from these recipes are so amazing you won't even realize you're eating healthy food. As we're nearing the end of this journey together, please honor yourself and take time and spend some time thinking about what this journey has meant to you so that you can apply what you've learned about longevity.

Afterword

I can't believe we've already reached the end of our journey together! Before we recap everything we've learned so far, and look at the next steps, I want to tell you one last story quickly.

After my trip to Italy and research on Italian health, I started implementing most of these principles in my life. At first, it didn't feel like it was making a difference, but one day I was faced with my progress and truly realized how far I've come. A few months after my work trip to Italy, I had a meeting with a colleague I would share the lecture stage with the following day. This day, I was the one on time, waiting for him in the lobby. As he came sprinting towards me across the room, I saw probably exactly what I looked like to the Italian doctor in Rome. The poor guy had run out of the hotel elevator, his tie barely around his neck and with his hands holding a paper coffee cup that was long empty. He held his laptop in his other hand and looked totally flustered. I saw an opportunity then to do for this doctor what that Italian doctor did for me: Introduce him to the Italian way of living.

Afterword

I invited him to sit down, and soon, we started chatting about work and life. I told him about the Italian longevity research I was busy with, and he was incredibly fascinated. I have no idea whether he applied the principles after he left the meeting. However, that's not in my control. All I can do is share my knowledge; the rest is up to you! My friend, this journey together has been incredible, but now it's your turn to take responsibility and act. It's up to you whether you want to forget all of what we just spoke about or whether you want to embrace it and change your health game completely.

You might initially feel a little overwhelmed or even uncomfortable, and that's normal. The important thing is that you take small steps at a time. So, how do we start living like Italians today? Well, let's start at the beginning.

- First, we can inspect our eating habits and identify areas we can improve. We can start being intentional with eating food that promotes longevity and try new recipes. Start making meals from scratch and visit your local farmer's market or organic food store for fresh ingredients. Add some new ingredients that you would usually avoid and try eating smaller portions. By doing these few things, your eating habits will already be significantly better than they used to be, creating space for you to live your best, healthiest life. Add some herbs you usually don't use and try experimenting with the Mediterranean diet a little more. Try growing your own herbs. Start small with basil, parsley, and oregano, and use your own fresh herbs in your recipes.
- Secondly, we can be intentional with staying active. Whether it's through going to the gym or starting a

post-dinner walk to the park, be intentional with getting in movement. The best place for most people to begin is by walking whenever possible. Decide to take the stairs instead of the elevator. Ask a friend or a family member to walk with you every other day and see how it goes. While cooking, ask Alexa to play Andrea Boccelli songs and dance around the kitchen. Put away the phone and take a yoga class online. Remember to create opportunities to move especially if don't naturally move a lot during the day. If you're up for it, join a class where you get to be active, like water aerobics or dancing. Getting in more movement will help you to feel more energized, and it will help you to live a longer, fuller life.

- Next, we can start by being more family-oriented and making time for our friends. When you spend time with friends and family, your physical and mental health will improve and remain strong. So, let's make it a priority. Stop pushing back visits with friends and family and put it at the top of your list. Think about how the Italians live and try to be more intentional with sharing meals with others. Be sure that you join a community where people have similar interests and values as you do and spend a lot of time with those people. You can also begin by volunteering or by simply not working less overtime. Prioritize your family and remember to find that balance between work and personal life.

- Finally, we can start living the Italian way by doing more of what we love. Follow your passion. Don't leave the things you love doing for end-of-the-year vacations or for when everything else on your list is finished. Prioritize doing more of what you love and find joy in the small moments of life. Enjoy resting and doing nothing, and remember to stop and smell the flowers and look at the stars. Doing what you love is what makes life worth all the ups and downs. Decide to live a sweet, peaceful life with less distraction. Live at a slower pace and start implementing the less is more rule.

Living the Italian way doesn't have to be complicated, but it does take being intentional with your time. It requires you to take some time to rest and be less productive in the eyes of the world. Also, remember that you have all this knowledge for a reason.

I can hear the objections from where I sit. I hate vegetables, I don't have time to cook, and I don't have time to exercise. I'm too tired after a long day of work. My family needs my full attention. My relatives drive me crazy - I can't spend time with them. The list is long and deep.

But take a step back and ask yourself - what prompted this book in the first place? My guess is that your curiosity was piqued by the fact that Italy has consistently had the healthiest people in the world, and this year in 2023, they are #1 in terms of health and wellness. Don't rationalize by thinking it's all genetics - the same Italian genes from immigrant parents and grandparents who were healthy in Italy generations ago now reside in Italian Americans who are suffering from every metabolic disease the American way of life offers. Many Italian Americans today truly resemble the television stereotypes of Italians.

There is something about the Italian way of life that works. There is a powerful saying I live by that I learned many years ago. It is "If you keep doing what you have been doing, you are going to keep getting what you have been getting"! If you want to help yourself live a longer and more fulfilled life, and you feel you are far from that mark, then it is time to *do something different.*

When you're unsure how to go about change, don't be afraid to go back and re-read the sections you're still struggling with. Before we say goodbye, let's recap everything we've discussed and discovered on this journey.

- We explored what it means to live the Italian way and looked at how Italians are the healthiest people on earth.
- We looked at the different blue zones and what it means to have blue zone status.
- We explored the Mediterranean diet and why it's so effective. We also looked at how the Italians have their own twist on the Mediterranean diet.
- We discovered that Italy has a strong food culture, including fresh and healthy foods, wine, and coffee.
- The Italians live the slow food movement, which is something we can all incorporate. The slow food movement is all about fresh food that is sourced ethically and taking the time to enjoy the blessings that food brings.
- We looked at the importance of family and how family can contribute to living longer and being healthier.
- We looked at how Italians stay fit and healthy and how their traditions contribute to their overall well-being.
- Finally, we looked at some recipes to help us on our journey.

Afterword

There is only one thing left to do. Are you ready to embrace the Italian lifestyle? Let's start living *La Dolce Vita and La Dolce Far Niente* and experience the sweetness of life and the joy of doing everything and nothing in life for ourselves, the Italian way.

Bibliography

Altomare, A. (2019, September 3). *The Italian Mediterranean Diet.* La Cucina Italiana. https://www.lacucinaitaliana.com/trends/healthy-food/italian-mediterranean-diet

Bartalesi, V. (2023, February 1). *Wine in Italian Culture—Why is it so Important?* Marronaia. https://www.marronaia.com/blog/wine-in-italian-culture-why-its-so-important/

Bensalhia, J. (2016, March 30). *10 Basics of Italian Food Culture You Need To Know.* Italy Magazine. https://www.italymagazine.com/featured-story/10-basics-italian-food-culture-you-need-know

Bezzone, F. (2019, October 30). *The History of Italian Cuisine I.* Life in Italy. https://lifeinitaly.com/the-history-of-italian-cuisine-i/

Bolla, N. (2020, September 16). *Working time in Italy: National Rules, Regulations and habits.* Accounting Bolla. https://accountingbolla.com/blog/working-time-in-italy-what-is-it-like-to-be-a-worker-in-modern-italy/

Brittney. (2022, November 1). *Dolce Far Niente: The Art of Doing Nothing.* Neveazzurra. https://www.neveazzurra.org/dolce-far-niente-the-art-of-doing-nothing/

Brown, L. (2022, December 21). *Which are the healthiest countries in the world for 2023?* CEO World Magazine. https://ceoworld.biz/2022/12/21/which-are-the-healthiest-countries-the-world-2023/

Buettner, D. (2008a). *Loma Linda, California.* Blue Zones. https://www.bluezones.com/explorations/loma-linda-california/

Buettner, D. (2008b). *Nicoya, Costa Rica.* Blue Zones. https://www.bluezones.com/explorations/nicoya-costa-rica/

Buettner, D. (2008c). *Okinawa, Japan.* Blue Zones. https://www.bluezones.com/explorations/okinawa-japan/

Capatti, A., & Montanari, M. (2016, October 15). *Italian Cuisine: A Cultural History.* Tuscany Cooking Class. https://blog.tuscany-cooking-class.com/regional-diversity-in-italian-cuisine/

Chandler, M. (2022, September 19). *An Exploration of Blue Zones and Human Longevity.* Thorne. https://www.thorne.com/take-5-daily/article/the-deep-dive-an-exploration-of-blue-zones-and-human-longevity

Change your habits—What You Can Do. (2022). Slow Food International. https://www.slowfood.com/what-we-do/themes/food-and-health/what-you-can-do/change-your-habits/

Bibliography

Characteristics of Work Culture in Italy. (2022). Italia Mia. https://www.italiamia.com/culture/characteristics-of-work-culture-in-italy/

Dombrowski, J. (2015, February 23). *8 Types of Italian Coffees, Explained.* Luxe Adventure Traveler. https://luxeadventuretraveler.com/types-of-italian-coffees/

8 Reasons why friendships are important for seniors. (2023). Amica Senior Living. https://www.amica.ca/conversations/8-reasons-why-friendships-are-important-for-seniors

Evason, N. (2017). *Italian Culture—Family.* Cultural Atlas. https://culturalatlas.sbs.com.au/italian-culture/italian-culture-family

Exploring Italian Cuisine: Flavorful Regions and a Fresh Perspective. (2019). Table Agent. https://tableagent.com/article/exploring-italian-cuisine-flavorful-regions-and-a-fresh-perspective/

Hengel, L. (2017, June 12). *Why Do Italians Live Longer Than the Rest of Europe?* The Culture Trip. https://theculturetrip.com/europe/italy/articles/italy-has-europes-oldest-population-why-the-longevity/

The History of Wine in Italy & Italian Wine Regions. (2021, October 21). Windstar Cruises Travel Blog. https://blog.windstarcruises.com/italy-wine-history/

Hutt, R. (2017, April 18). *Italy may have a struggling economy but its people are the healthiest in the world.* World Economic Forum. https://www.weforum.org/agenda/2017/04/italy-may-have-a-struggling-economy-but-its-people-are-the-healthiest-on-earth/

Ikaria, Greece. (n.d.). Blue Zones. Retrieved May 18, 2023, from https://www.bluezones.com/explorations/ikaria-greece/

Katira, K. (2022). *Four secrets to longevity from the centenarians of Okinawa, the land of immortals.* WION News. https://www.wionews.com/entertainment/lifestyle/news-_-secrets-to-longevity-from-the-centenarians-of-okinawa-537851

Ledsom, A. (2022, May 4). *Why Are People Living Longer in One Italian Village?* Forbes. https://www.forbes.com/sites/alexledsom/2022/05/04/why-are-people-living-longer-in-one-italian-village/?sh=119701 8b2f12

Lorne Blyth. (2016, July 5). *How Food Plays a Part in an Everyday Italian Lifestyle & Culture.* Flavours Holidays. https://www.flavoursholidays.co.uk/blog/food-in-italian-lifestyle/

Ludwig, D. (2017, January 31). *Try This 15-Minute After-Dinner Ritual That Helps Italians Lose Weight.* Prevention. https://www.prevention.com/weight-loss/a20503013/try-this-15-minute-after-dinner-ritual-that-helps-italians-lose-weight/

Mason, S. (2023). 40+ Shocking Fast Food Statistics For 2023 | US & Worldwide Data. *Eat Pallet.* https://eatpallet.com/fast-food-statistics/

Bibliography

McGuire, G. (2017, July 11). *Welcome to Acciaroli, the Italian Village Where Residents Live Into Their 100s.* Culture Trip. https://theculturetrip.com/europe/italy/articles/welcome-to-acciaroli-the-italian-village-where-residents-live-into-their-100s/

Mediterranean Diet. (2022, November 20). Cleveland Clinic. https://my.clevelandclinic.org/health/articles/16037-mediterranean-diet

Meleen, M. (2021, September 21). *Why Is Family Important? 9 Reasons It Benefits Us (and Society).* Love to Know. https://www.lovetoknow.com/life/lifestyle/why-is-family-important

Mikhail, A. (2023, April 2). *The secrets to longevity that help residents of America's only blue zone city live healthier and longer lives.* Fortune Well. https://fortune.com/well/2023/04/02/longevity-tips-loma-linda-california-blue-zone-city/

Miles, G. (2020, May 22). *What the Healthiest Countries in the World Have in Common.* Toronto Tribune. https://www.thetorontotribune.com/2020/05/22/what-the-healthiest-countries-in-the-world-have-in-common/

The Nutrition Source. (2018, December 12). *Diet Review: Mediterranean Diet.* Harvard School of Public Health. https://www.hsph.harvard.edu/nutrition-source/healthy-weight/diet-reviews/mediterranean-diet/

Our philosophy—About us. (2015). Slow Food International. https://www.slowfood.com/about-us/our-philosophy/

Pitura, P. (2021, October 6). *Blue Zone Costa Rica: Living Longer, Living Better.* Special Places of Costa Rica. https://www.specialplacesofcostarica.com/blue-zone-costa-rica-living-longer-living-better/

Prentice, M. (2020, December 15). *Traditions Passed Down Through Generations.* Italy Segreta. https://italysegreta.com/traditions-passed-down-through-generations/

Raman, R. (2018, July 14). *14 Healthy Whole Grain Foods (Including Gluten-Free Options).* Healthline. https://www.healthline.com/nutrition/whole-grain-foods

Russell, H. (2019, May 22). *Dolce far niente: Learn the Italian art of doing nothing.* The Globe and Mail. https://www.theglobeandmail.com/life/travel/article-dolce-far-niente-learn-the-italian-art-of-doing-nothing/

Salomon, S. H., & Lawler, M. (2022, June 10). *8 Scientific Health Benefits of the Mediterranean Diet.* Everyday Health. https://www.everydayhealth.com/mediterranean-diet/scientific-health-benefits-mediterranean-diet/

Sardinian Tomato Salad. (2017, July 14). Martha Stewart. https://www.marthastewart.com/1518336/sardinian-tomato-salad

Sinadinou, E. (2018, December 6). *How to Live to 100: Lessons from the Blue Zone Island of Ikaria.* Greece Is. https://www.greece-is.com/how-to-live-to-100-lessons-from-the-blue-zone-island-of-ikaria/

Bibliography

Slow Food Movement Guide: Definition, History. (2021, September 5). Slow Living LDN. https://slowlivingldn.com/journal/live-consciously/what-is-the-slow-food-movement/

Spector, N. (2019, April 3). *What "Blue Zone" city Loma Linda, California can teach us about living longer*. NBC News. https://www.nbcnews.com/better/lifestyle/what-blue-zone-city-loma-linda-california-can-teach-us-ncna989661

Statistica; *Fast food restaurant sector market size US 2022 | Statista*. (2022, November 14). Statista. https://www.statista.com/statistics/1174417/fast-food-restaurants-industry-market-size-us/#:

A study on the longevity of Campodimele inhabitants. (n.d.). Britannica. Retrieved May 16, 2023, from https://www.britannica.com/video/179456/inhabitants-Researchers-longevity-Italy-Campodimele

Thatcher, T. (2020, March 17). *The Top 10 Benefits of Spending Time With Family*. Highland Springs. https://highlandspringsclinic.org/the-top-ten-benefits-of-spending-time-with-family/

Thomas, A. (2022, July 1). *The Strong Knot of Italian Friendship*. Italy Segreta. https://italysegreta.com/the-strong-knot-of-italian-friendship/

Thomas, A. J. (2022). *Italian Family Life: A Look at the Culture*. Love to Know. https://www.lovetoknow.com/life/relationships/italian-family-life

Tucci, C. (2020, July 27). *How to Live to 100: Lessons From Italy*. Lifespan. https://www.lifespan.org/lifespan-living/how-live-100-lessons-italy

Why Do Italians Live So Long? (2019, April 1). Contento Italiano. https://contentoitaliano.com/why-italians-live-so-long/

Image References

Christiaans, F. (2022, February 24). [*Italian Vineyard*] [Image]. Unsplash. https://unsplash.com/photos/4BuDJxjJ9ys

Curry, C. (2020, April 27). [*Italian Coastal Town*] [Image]. Unsplash. https://unsplash.com/photos/HzoICgtDEds

Du Preez, P. (2018, June 10). [*People Eating Together*] [Image]. Unsplash. https://unsplash.com/photos/W3SEyZODn8U

Dumlao, N. (2017, October 26). [*Coffee*] [Image]. Unsplash. https://unsplash.com/photos/zUNs99PGDgo

Fernández, N. (2020, April 9). [*Nicoya Peninsula*] [Image]. Unsplash. https://unsplash.com/photos/LV7B8KN3F28

Filatova, N. (2020, May 11). [*Traditional Pizza*] [Image]. Unsplash. https://unsplash.com/photos/frTrM7Gdkho

Gan, C. (2016, March 22). [*Pasta*] [Image]. Unsplash. https://unsplash.com/photos/KSXvrqKUxnc

Bibliography

Gionfriddo, M. (2020, June 30). [*Italian Cafe*] [Image]. Unsplash. https://unsplash.com/photos/II3Vo7MJ9Zo

Gottardi, C. (2017, August 29). [*Old People Happy*] [Image]. Unsplash. https://unsplash.com/photos/6Frs5Cht6Pc

JW. (2019, March 2). [*Old People Walking*] [Image]. Unsplash. https://unsplash.com/photos/zmMtb3PtsrE

Kabajev, A. (2020, October 19). [*Old Besties*] [Image]. Unsplash. https://unsplash.com/photos/_aduPjJvDx4

Kallergis, L. (2019, March 23). [*Red Wine*] [Image]. Unsplash. https://unsplash.com/photos/etWlaoFnTl4

Kavvadas, N. (2018, August 1). [*Italian Farmer's Market*] [Image]. Unsplash. https://unsplash.com/photos/sYMvH-4AB_Q

Lark, B. (2017, February 1). [*Mediterranean Food*] [Image]. Unsplash. https://unsplash.com/photos/C1fMH2Vej8A

May, G. (2020, January 4). [*Ikaria*] [Image]. Unsplash. https://unsplash.com/photos/9UoqqoqKEOc

Pallian, J. (2017, February 1). [*Mediterranean Fish*] [Image]. Unsplash. https://unsplash.com/photos/8pUjhBm4cLw

Peralta, H. (2020, August 3). [*Old Lady*] [Image]. Unsplash. https://unsplash.com/photos/dtgSAJVSqv8

Sho, K. (2021, January 18). [*Okinawa*] [Image]. Unsplash. https://unsplash.com/photos/1twczdE1zlE

Sorge, R. (2016, September 27). [*Olive Oil*] [Image]. Unsplash. https://unsplash.com/photos/uOBApnN_K7w

Virgilio, M. (2020, November 13). [*Sardinia*] [Image]. Unsplash. https://unsplash.com/photos/iSORmTk3pao

Author's Notes

Dear Reader,

I would like to thank you for purchasing this book and taking the time to read through the material. I hope you enjoyed reading it as much as I enjoyed writing it, and my sincere wish is that you take from it a new understanding of the health, wellness, and happiness that can be yours. The Secrets of Italian Self Care was a joy for me to write and share. My roots are Italian, and this book has been my homecoming! I hope that it is yours also.

I would like to take this time to humbly ask that you leave an honest review on Amazon or on whatever platform you purchased this book, as I do take the time to read all of them. The reviews help me in my own personal growth, and they assist me in making improvements to my published works. Your review will help others find what this book offers, and that help will be greatly appreciated. I extend my sincerest gratitude for your time. May we all find the best of health and wellness in our lives and achieve our fullest potential.

Author's Notes

Please follow this link to leave a review on your Amazon Account:

https://www.amazon.com/review/create-review/?asin= BoC88XPSZ1.

Thank you!

Yours in good health,

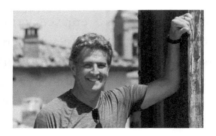

Dr. Gene Antenucci

Made in United States
Troutdale, OR
07/25/2023

11557075R00080